# 3 WEEKS
# TO A BETTER BACK

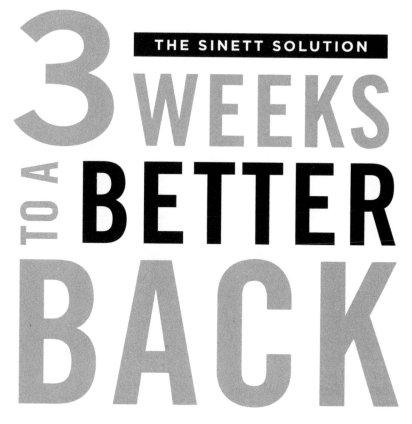

**THE SINETT SOLUTION**

# 3 WEEKS TO A BETTER BACK

Solutions for Healing the Structural, Nutritional, and Emotional Causes of Back Pain

## DR. TODD SINETT

**EAST
END
PRESS**

Published by
EAST END PRESS
Bridgehampton, NY

Library of Congress Control Number: 2015948119

ISBN 978-0-9887673-8-6
Ebook ISBN 978-0-9887673-9-3

FIRST EDITION

Book Design by Elyse Strongin, Neuwirth & Associates
Jacket Design by Dave Reidy

Manufactured in the United States of America

10  9  8  7  6  5  4  3  2  1

*To my dad who had the courage to be different. He left me with large shoes to fill but thankfully enough of a footprint, so that I can continue what he started. I truly hope this book helps you live a happier and healthier life.*

# CONTENTS

# How Much Do You *Really* Know About Back Pain?

## Take this quiz and find out just how knowledgeable you are!

1. Where does back pain rank in caused missed work days? First, second, third, or fourth?

2. How helpful are MRIs in the diagnosis of back pain?
   - a. Absolutely a must for any back pain sufferer.
   - b. A complete waste of money
   - c. Mildly helpful
   - d. Potentially harmful
   - e. Two of the above

3. Proper bending and lifting techniques are vital to prevent back pain.
   - a. True
   - b. False

4. What you eat and drink can be the cause of your back pain.
   - a. False
   - b. True, too much sugar and alcohol are the culprits.
   - c. True, too much salad and roughage are to blame.
   - d. Two of the above

5. Sit-ups and crunches are a good way to strengthen your abs and thus stabilize your back.
   - a. There is no relation between your ab function and your back.
   - b. The more crunches and sit-ups you do the better.
   - c. Sit-ups and crunches have nothing to do with stabilizing your back.
   - d. You shouldn't do a sit-up, but crunches are okay.

6. If you have a disc herniation there is nothing that you can do—except live with the pain.
   - a. True
   - b. False

7. The key to ridding yourself of back pain is:
    a. A good stretch regimen
    b. A good surgeon
    c. A good chiropractor
    d. All or none of the above

8. The phrase, "Lose the weight, lose the back pain" is:
    a. An oversimplified model
    b. For the most part true
    c. Weight and back pain don't correlate.
    d. None of the above

9. Surgery is a good long-term solution to back pain.
    a. True
    b. False
    c. You have got to be crazy to have back surgery.
    d. It can be, but use it as a last option.

10. You can exercise your way out of back pain.
    a. True
    b. False
    c. Rest is best when you suffer from back pain.
    d. Take some aspirin or Tylenol and do it anyway.

11. The number one predictor of back pain is:
    a. Low flexibility
    b. Stress and emotional outlook
    c. Diet
    d. Strength

12. The annual amount of money spent on back pain treatment and diagnosis in The United States is around:
    a. $10 billion
    b. $850 million
    c. $25 billion
    d. $80 billion

13. The best way to sit is:
    a. Up straight
    b. With a slight slouch forward
    c. Slightly angled backward
    d. None of the above

14. Regular care (such as chiropractic, massage, and physical therapy), exercise, eating right, and stress management is the best way to stay free of back pain.
    a. True
    b. False
    c. Back pain is inevitable anyway
    d. Back pain is genetic

15. Back pain can be:
    a. A sign of a significant medical emergency
    b. A mild annoyance
    c. A cause of a significant disability
    d. The greatest thing that ever happened to you
    e. All of the above

---

Flip to page 237 to see how many questions you got right. If you answered some questions incorrectly, that's okay! This book will help you better understand the body and the back, so that you can test and feel 100% after reading!

# INTRODUCTION

"All truths are easy to understand once they are discovered.
The point is to discover them."

—GALILEO GALILEI

Since you're reading this book, I feel it's safe to assume that you are suffering from back pain. I also assume that whatever you have been doing to treat your back pain hasn't worked. Let's be honest, who reads a book about back pain if they've already found relief? This book contains my solution to most types of back pain—and my solution will become your solution. I can promise you it won't be overly technical.

It doesn't matter whether back pain plagues you daily or occasionally, has been creeping in or seems to have struck out the blue. If back pain is interfering with your life, now you have become a statistic. Yes. A statistic. That's because 20% of the population is currently suffering from back pain, and 85% of people will suffer from it at some point.

Here are some other shocking truths I've found:

- ▶ In April 2014, back pain became the number one reason people around the world took disability from work.

- ▶ Back pain is second only to the common cold as the reason people visit their doctors.

- ▶ Back pain is the third most common reason for hospitalization.

- ▶ It is the fifth most common cause for surgery.

- ▶ 33% percent of all people over the age of 18 have sought treatment for back pain in the last five years.

▶ Our healthcare system spends upwards of $80 billion on the diagnosis and treatment of back pain.

All these statistics lead to the obvious but concerning conclusion that back pain is a natural occurrence, and we need to learn how to cope with it. The majority of sufferers feel their back pain is inescapable and have resigned themselves to living with it. Even the most well-intentioned doctors often have you believing this inevitable reality and prescribe pain-killers to help you get by.

To me, the stats represent a dismal failure—the failure of our doctors in diagnosing and treating back pain. These stats are screaming for a completely different approach. The Sinett Solution is that completely different approach.

The truth about back pain is that you are still suffering because your doctor is only looking at your back. This means he or she is missing the source of your pain and has been misdiagnosing you. Proper back pain treatment is all about finding the correct root of the problem—and often, the problem is not where the pain is. Back pain *can* be structural, right in the back, but it is most often caused by an imbalance elsewhere in the body, in your digestion or emotions. Yes, that's right. For most, the problem is not your back. It's your feet, your shoulders, your core, your stress, and your diet. It's the little choices that you have been making over time that have slowly been crippling the systems of your body, which are all impacted and manifest through the spine, the body's great connector. If you have received back treatment and are still suffering, that's because your pain may not be coming from your back.

The Sinett Solution is a three-pronged, three-week simple approach to getting rid of back pain by targeting the points of the body and mind that you have been ignoring. As I said, the current model of treatment typically only addresses the structural issues in the discs and muscles of the back—but that ignores the rest of your body! The correct strategy for most means targeting a combination of structural, digestive, and emotional issues. First, you must figure out what type of back pain sufferer you are and where your pain is stemming from. You need to properly self-diagnose the problem by examining your total body as well as your back. An incomplete or incorrect diagnosis will lead to improper treatments and suffering. Once you arrive at a correct diagnosis, you can treat your pain in just three weeks. This book will give you the tools to correctly self-diagnose and formulate a strategy to treat your particular type of back pain.

When you're looking to uncover the root of your pain, you must remember to keep in mind that your body has its own language. It is communicating specifically through posture, pain, and tension. Up until now, most of you have probably ignored your body's messages and may even have attempted to quiet or shut off the body's language with pain medications that cover up the pain, rather than getting to the root of it. If you don't listen to the signs and symptoms your body is sending you, you will miss the glaring clues which can result in an incorrect diagnosis. I often hear, "My back pain just came out of nowhere!" Unless you had a fall or an accident, this is impossible! Your back pain certainly is coming from somewhere, and you probably weren't aware enough of your body's language to recognize the precursor to the pain!

The Sinett Solution starts with your very own Inflammatory (BPI) score. Your score will tell you where your back pain is coming from. By identifying the way your body is directing its stress and inflammation and determining the source of your pain, you can tailor a solution to fit your particular problem. Then, by following the appropriate treatment that I recommend to alleviate the pain, you will feel results in just three weeks. That is the truth—and once you find the correct approach to treating your particular pain, you will wonder why it took you so long to discover something so simple.

## THE START TO THE SINETT SOLUTION

When people first hear my theory, they immediately understand how back pain can be caused by a structural problem—a trauma to the body, poor posture, even too much sitting at your computer desk. But they wonder, *how can back pain be emotional or digestive?* It doesn't make sense right away, but it became really easy for me to understand when my father, a practicing chiropractor, found himself crippled with back pain that wasn't eased with the typical chiropractic treatment.

For 15 years, my father worked from eight in the morning until eight at night, seeing patient after patient, until one day, he bent down to pick up a tennis ball but could not get up. "I threw my back out," he said and took a few days off from work to rest in bed. But the days turned into weeks, and the weeks turned into nine long months without any relief from his spasms and pain.

For those nine months, my father searched for answers to his own back problem. He went for endless treatments and consultations with every known profession, including his own, but nothing helped. A surgeon recommended exploratory surgery (never a good option), offering to open him up to see if they could find anything.

Hoping to find another option, he went to see a doctor in Detroit with the fortuitous name of Dr. George Goodheart who asked one question that no one else had bothered to ask: *Why are you having back spasms?* All the other doctors failed to come up with a successful treatment because they focused only on treating the spasms rather than finding out what was causing them. According to Dr. Goodheart, the answer, oddly enough, was that my father's diet, which consisted of sugar and caffeine, was upsetting his digestive system. Anything that can upset your digestive system can then reflex, inflame, and impact your muscular system, thus causing back spasms, according to this doctor. My father's reaction to this concept was complete disbelief. But given that his only options were to either change his diet or have exploratory surgery, he chose to change his diet. Dr. Goodheart treated him just a few times in conjunction with a complete change in his nutrition, and lo and behold, my father was cured in a few short weeks.

My father's life and my family's lives were changed forever. The problem was not his back! My father dedicated his professional time to learning and expanding the teachings of Dr. Goodheart. This unique physician often spoke of the triad of health, or bringing one's body into balance on three different levels:

1. Structural, or treating problems in the muscle, bones or nerves.
2. Digestive, determining the effects of your diet and nutrition, as well as toxins and hormones.
3. Emotional, understanding the impact of stress and the way it manifests in physical pain.

At the core of this theory is the idea that all parts of the body are connected. Armed with this new knowledge and approach, my father became quite successful in treating pain in thousands of patients. I joined him in this practice after having my own pivotal experience. It was my sophomore year in college, and I was unsure of what to do in my life. We were on vacation in Aruba, and the local pediatrician had asked my father if he would examine a boy who was suffering from debilitating headaches. I went along with my dad to the local hospital and watched as he found that the boy's headaches were coming from an imbalance in his jaw and cranial bones. My father gave him one treatment, and the boy's headache went away.

I knew from that day on that I would join my father and learn more about back pain because I believed that there were very few people in the world who could have helped that boy. Plenty of doctors had already failed. My father said it actually wasn't that complicated—he just looked at the patient differently. He saw when the problem wasn't the patient's back.

After witnessing the boy's recovery and his family's deepest gratitude, I realized I was being handed both a gift and a responsibility: to help people and to change the way the world views and treats back pain. I knew I had to find a successful treatment that I could offer to many more people than just those who walk through my practice doors. By applying what I know about the triad of health, I've discovered that back pain is often easier to treat on your own, without a doctor, in just three weeks.

## Why three weeks? Is that enough?

Yes! The source of your back pain can be identified by quickly understanding what works and what does not. And because our back pain is caused by some combination of digestive issues, emotional stress, and the physical strain of everyday activities like sitting (yes, sitting! Sitting has even been labeled "the new smoking!"), very often the key to ridding yourself of back pain is changing unhealthy habits into healthy ones. Research has shown that changing a habit or creating a new healthy one takes about 21 days. If you try something and you don't see an improvement in three weeks, you haven't found your "truth" and you need to listen more closely to your body's language. However, I'm confident my approach to self-diagnosis will help you get it right the first time so you're able to determine the exact source of your pain.

## What does a self-treatment strategy entail?

Depending on whether your pain is structural, digestive, or emotional, we can effectively correct your imbalances, modify your eating habits, and even change your stress response with our Enerchi techniques in just three weeks. I will provide all of the exercises, recipes, and nutrition options, as well as a variety of stress-reducing strategies to help you formulate the right plan for your specific needs. Remember, the systems of the body are interconnected, so your solution will likely have components of all three!

Now that I have discovered a successful method to diagnosing and treating back pain, the truth is easy to understand! Back pain is curable, often without surgery and pain medication, and my solution will help you return to optimal function in three weeks.

So what do you have to lose? (Besides your back pain!)

*   *   *

I AM A *testament to the Sinett Solution. I was referred to Dr. Sinett by my girlfriend, who had been pitching Dr. Sinett to me for months. I was hesitant and actually urged by my doctors not to seek out alternative care; however, the decision to seek alternative medicine has turned out to be the most beneficial decision I have made. My case, while not just your typical back pain case, is a lesson on how important it is to adopt the Sinett Solution approach.*

*I grew up in a small town in Canada, and like most Canadian kids immediately fell in love with hockey. I played junior hockey, subsequently earning a scholarship to college, getting one step closer to my dream of playing professionally. That dream ended after I took a hit which caused a concussion. As a result of that hit, I suffered from severe headaches and neck pain that lasted for many years. I was going to neurologists and orthopedists, but the treatments they were providing did not bring any relief. Not only were they not helping, their advice was to simply lay low and let the symptoms run their course. As time went on, it became clearer that their ultimate message was that I should get used to a life consumed with headaches.*

*I can't begin to tell you how much I was suffering. I begrudgingly went to Dr. Sinett, and the first thing he saw was how tight my jaw was. He explained that my jaw had been seriously impacted from the check and subsequent whiplash. He also found that my posture and core were way off balance. Dr. Sinett pointed out that I had spent more than 20 years hunched over a hockey stick and then a few years hunched over my computer monitor. Perhaps it was common sense, but it was not something I would have realized would cause such a headache! Also, my training involved thousands of crunches to help get my core strong, which helped compound the symptoms. Dr. Sinett explained that all of this forward* pull was putting tremendous strain on my neck and shoulders and could be causing my headaches and pain. He started me on his Backbridge™ and at the beginning I could barely lay on level 1; in a couple of months, I was able to lay on all five levels.

Dr. Sinett also discovered that my body still seemed quite tight and inflamed so we looked into my diet. Being Canadian, I really like my beer, but after analyzing my diet, we decided to eliminate it for a few weeks. I couldn't believe what a difference this made. Thankfully, I have been able to switch to whiskey without it aggravating my symptoms; it is a nice substitute and something I never would have thought of myself. Dr. Sinett also discussed the role that my stress was having on my condition, and as a result I have really become tuned in when my stress triggers my muscular tension.

Dr. Sinett and his approach has really changed my life. He now has me doing some PT to work on my flexibility and posture which is working really well where the previous PT recommended by other doctors hadn't helped. I now know that my condition needs the structural, nutritional, and emotional systems to all be in balance for me to function optimally.

*Jared Keller*

# So You Think You Know Back Pain

# 1

# WHAT KIND OF SUFFERER ARE YOU?

## Defining Your Back Pain

"**M**y back hurts" sounds like a simple complaint, but it's actually your body pleading for attention. Patients often come to me with a variety of guesses as to what caused their pain: trauma or injury, degeneration of the vertebrae, protruding disc, ligament or muscle tears, muscle tension, overuse or improper exercise, poor muscle tone, back-related joint problems, obesity, etc. The list goes on and on. Even before attempting to diagnose the cause as structural, digestive, or emotional, it's important to understand how long you've been suffering, what you have done to try to help yourself, and if you haven't done anything, why that is.

In working with back pain patients for about 20 years, I have found that back pain sufferers fall into five different categories. While the treatments are uniquely based on the cause of their back pain, these five categories are distinguished by the patient's feelings and beliefs about their back and how they respond to pain. It is important to correctly categorize a sufferer for two reasons:

1. The categories allow the doctor to properly understand the patient and determine the most sensitive approach. Ultimately, communication with the patient must correctly match the corresponding category. Without this connection, the patient will end up having unrealistic expectations and conclusions.

2. The categories help the patient define his or her belief system about their pain and change his or her consciousness.

Why do you need to change your consciousness? Don't we just need to change your back? Well, a patient's beliefs about back pain are often the barrier to finding a permanent solution. You are not to blame. Your belief system about your back pain has come from the false assumptions our medical society has created. We as a society have made you believe that back pain is a natural progression of life and that everyone will and should learn to deal with it. The truth is there are treatment options that can help, no matter what kind of sufferer you are.

Below are my five categories of back pain sufferers and their harmful beliefs. By taking the Back Pain Sufferer Assessment, you will figure out in which category you may belong. Once this is accomplished, we can go to work fixing your belief system. If you can't correctly fix your belief system, you cannot be free of your back pain.

## BACK PAIN SUFFERER ASSESSMENT

### 1. THE QUIET MANAGER

**"A little pain is normal—everyone feels this way."**

*Answer "yes" or "no" to the following statements to determine if you are a Quiet Manager.*

|  | YES | NO |
|---|---|---|
| On a scale of 1 to 10, with 10 being the most severe and 0 being no pain, most days your back pain is between 1 and 3. | ☐ | ☐ |
| You need to take an over-the-counter anti-inflammatory for your back pain at least a few times a month. | ☐ | ☐ |
| You pay attention to sleeping in the proper position. | ☐ | ☐ |
| You can't sit too long and need to stand up and move around because your back starts to bother you. | ☐ | ☐ |
| You hesitate to lift things because you worry you may hurt your back. | ☐ | ☐ |
| You take an Advil, Tylenol, or other OTC painkillers in anticipation of playing sports. | ☐ | ☐ |
| You know that after an evening on your feet, your back is going to hurt the next day. | ☐ | ☐ |

|  | YES | NO |
|---|---|---|
| You haven't sought professional care or treatment for your back. | ☐ | ☐ |
| You have gone for treatment for your back but were told that you are essentially fine or you felt minimal improvement from the care. | ☐ | ☐ |
| You make sure that you bend properly. | ☐ | ☐ |
| Your back pain doesn't really stop you from doing the things that you want, but you are aware of it. | ☐ | ☐ |
| You avoid specific exercises or activities because you know it will hurt your back. | ☐ | ☐ |
| You don't bother mentioning your back pain to your loved ones because it is no big deal. | ☐ | ☐ |

*If you answered "yes" to three or more questions, you are a Quiet Manager.*

I would characterize the majority of back pain sufferers as quiet managers. You don't necessarily think you are suffering from back pain and won't seek out any treatment for what you believe to be "normal" aches and pains. But that's the sneaky thing about most back pain: it doesn't come from a traumatic event, such as a fall or car accident, but rather creeps up, little by little each day, sometimes so slowly that you don't even notice it. In most cases, it has been building for years, and now that you are aware of some discomfort, you typically associate it with growing older.

While you may not be as agile as you were a few years back, you shouldn't be simply accepting your pain as an inevitable part of aging. And yet you have become the quiet manager, a master of living around the limitations your back now imposes. You pay careful attention to sleeping in a certain way, not sitting too long, or not lifting things that are too heavy. You make sure you bend properly, and you may even perform back stretches religiously. If you over exert yourself, you take over-the-counter medication. In fact, you may even pop a few pills in anticipation of moderate exertion.

You are not aware how much your back is adversely affecting you. Only after we are able to help you feel better will you look back and realize how bad it was! The limiting belief factor for the quiet manager is that it is normal to suffer quietly. Resigning yourself to that fate is a mistake. You don't need to feel this way!

It's important for quiet managers to honestly assess their emotions and why you haven't spoken up about your pain. Ask yourself:

|  | YES | NO |
|---|---|---|
| Do I have other ailments I am "coping" with? | ☐ | ☐ |
| Do I bottle up my stress? | ☐ | ☐ |

When did I first notice the pain creeping in?  _____

Your tendency to ignore your pain is your harmful behavior, and the belief that pain is normal is where we need to change your consciousness. This book will help you listen to the small signs of your body, modify your unhealthy habits, and remind you why you deserve to be proactive about your health.

Quiet managers can also fall into another category of sufferer, so even if this category defines you, take the following quizzes and see if any other descriptions apply! Remember, total treatment is the only way to a cure, so finding all of your false beliefs and correcting them is the first step to a better life!

## 2. THE NON-TRAUMATIC ACUTE SUFFERER

**"My back went out. I will just load up on
some Tylenol and it will go away."**

*Answer "yes" or "no" to the following statements to determine if you are a Non-Traumatic Acute Sufferer.*

|  | YES | NO |
|---|---|---|
| Your back pain doesn't consistently bother you but you have had bouts of pain that were higher than a 6 on a scale of 1 to 10 and lasted from one to two days up to two weeks. | ☐ | ☐ |
| You bent over and your back "went out." | ☐ | ☐ |
| You believe that your severe back pain came out of nowhere. | ☐ | ☐ |
| You woke up one morning and were either barely able to turn your head or could barely stand up straight. | ☐ | ☐ |

|  | YES | NO |
|---|---|---|
| You got a severe back pain after catching a draft. | ☐ | ☐ |
| You have missed days from work because of your back pain. | ☐ | ☐ |
| For women, the pain came on right around your menstrual cycle. | ☐ | ☐ |
| You load up on the pain relievers, whether they are over-the-counter or prescription, just to help deal with the immediate pain. | ☐ | ☐ |
| Simple movements such as getting dressed or tying your shoes are quite difficult. | ☐ | ☐ |
| You are bent over in pain. | ☐ | ☐ |
| You started a new diet, new vitamin, or new medication. | ☐ | ☐ |
| Your stomach has recently been bothering you. | ☐ | ☐ |
| You have recently been constipated or had diarrhea. | ☐ | ☐ |
| You recently had too much alcohol or spicy food. | ☐ | ☐ |

*Answer "yes" to three or more of these issues? You are a Non-Traumatic Acute Sufferer.*

If you fall into this category, you have pain caused by something non-impactful, meaning you weren't hit by a car or didn't fall off your bike. Maybe one day you slept funny or lifted wrong and your back or neck "went out." This acute pain is your opportunity because pain is a great motivator to seek help. Unfortunately, our methods for treatment for back pain are so poor that the vast majority of acute-pain patients hear a similar diagnosis ("It isn't anything serious!") and receive a superficial treatment ("Try a few anti-inflammatories, maybe stretch a bit—you should be fine"). Often, the pain eventually lessens back to a "manageable" level—until the next episode and the vicious, unnecessary cycle occurs all over again. This is because there is something bigger going on, causing these attacks to recur throughout your life. Often the non-traumatic acute sufferer is a regular quiet sufferer.

If you feel you fall into the category of Non-Traumatic Acute Sufferer, it's important that you recall previous times when you've experienced a similar type of back pain and remember what was going on in your life at that time.

|                                                                      | YES | NO |
|----------------------------------------------------------------------|-----|-----|
| Were you eating poorly?                                              | ☐   | ☐  |
| Were you in a life transition (a new job, new home, break-up, etc.)? | ☐   | ☐  |
| Do you have a tendency to fall in and out of the same bad habits?   | ☐   | ☐  |

With the Non-Traumatic Sufferer, it's important to change the belief that the pain came out of nowhere. You didn't just bend wrong. The pain, rather, has been building little by little and a simple movement was more like the straw that broke the camel's back rather than the cause. You need to believe and understand this so that we can detect the true source of your pain, which could even be diet or stress. The Sinett Solution will help you arrive at the deeper root of that pain and find permanent relief. Remember, your Tylenol is only giving you six hours of it!

## 3. THE CHRONIC SUFFERER

### "I have a bad back and I will just deal with it."

*Answer "yes" or "no" to the following statements to determine if you are a Chronic Sufferer.*

|                                                                                                                          | YES | NO |
|--------------------------------------------------------------------------------------------------------------------------|-----|-----|
| On a scale of 1 to 10, with 10 being the most severe and 0 being no pain, most days your back pain is between a 4 and 7. | ☐   | ☐  |
| You frequently take an over-the-counter medication to help you deal with your back pain.                                 | ☐   | ☐  |
| It is a rare occurrence if your back doesn't bother you in a day.                                                        | ☐   | ☐  |
| You don't lift your young children because of your back pain.                                                            | ☐   | ☐  |
| You pretty much have back pain all of the time.                                                                         | ☐   | ☐  |
| You are hard-pressed to remember a day when your back wasn't an issue.                                                   | ☐   | ☐  |
| Your stomach frequently bothers you.                                                                                    | ☐   | ☐  |
| You regularly feel gassy.                                                                                               | ☐   | ☐  |

|  | YES | NO |
|---|---|---|
| You take pain medication (either prescription or over-the-counter) on a regular/frequent basis. | ☐ | ☐ |
| You frequently suffer from constipation or diarrhea. | ☐ | ☐ |
| You generally have a poor diet that may contain high levels of sugars, caffeine, or alcohol. | ☐ | ☐ |
| You have quite a repetitive diet, tending to eat the same food over and over again. | ☐ | ☐ |
| You tend to be food sensitive to groups such as gluten or dairy. | ☐ | ☐ |
| You believe that you have a bad back. | ☐ | ☐ |

*Did one of these questions get a "yes"? If so, you are a Chronic Sufferer.*

The Chronic Sufferer experiences "unmanageable" back pain for a prolonged period of time, and he believes he or she just has to find a way to cope. Prolonged back pain really takes a toll on your quality of life. Perhaps you are considering surgery, or have even had it but it did not help. You have tried seemingly everything but nothing has worked. The longer you suffer from pain, the more you believe it will never go away.

The Chronic Sufferer more likely suffers from poor medical care than his or her true medical condition. The Chronic Sufferer needs to be open to try some new things and ask:

What has provided you with some relief other than painkillers?

_____

_____

_____

_____

_____

_____

_____

|                                                                                              | YES | NO |
|----------------------------------------------------------------------------------------------|-----|----|
| Would you consider yourself a good eater? Have you simultaneously suffered digestive upsets?  | ☐   | ☐  |
| Do you feel like you deal well with your stress?                                             | ☐   | ☐  |

If you are open to something new, there is still hope! Even if you have chronic pain, some of my very simple solutions will be able to alleviate your pain. To me, the length of time that you have been suffering is not an indicative factor of the seriousness of your condition, but more an indictment of how ineffective your prior treatments have been. This book discusses both the causes of chronic back pain as well as solutions that you usually won't hear about from other physicians.

## 4. THE LIFE-SENTENCE SUFFERER

**"There is nothing that can be done other than surgery.
If that doesn't help, I'm stuck in pain forever."**

*Answer "yes" or "no" to the following statements to determine if you are a Life-Sentence Sufferer.*

|                                                                                       | YES | NO |
|---------------------------------------------------------------------------------------|-----|----|
| You have had an MRI and been diagnosed with a herniated disc.                          | ☐   | ☐  |
| You have been diagnosed with spinal stenosis, degenerative disc disease, or arthritis. | ☐   | ☐  |
| You have had surgery and still have back pain.                                         | ☐   | ☐  |
| You have tried everything but nothing has helped.                                     | ☐   | ☐  |
| You take prescription medication to help you deal with your back.                      | ☐   | ☐  |

*Did you rack up at least one "yes"? You are a Life-Sentence sufferer.*

The Chronic Sufferer and the Life-Sentence Sufferer will present very similarly; however the main difference is that the Life-Sentence Sufferer has been branded with a condition that becomes a prescription for a lifetime of suffering. You may have had some testing, such as an MRI, which confirmed this sentence with a diagnosis of arthritis, degenerative disc disease, herniated discs, or spinal stenosis. The results of the tests leave you convinced that your pain is never going to go away!

These back pain patients tend to have the deepest belief system because they are convinced—even by their doctors—that they must suffer forever. But Life-Sentence sufferers, I have news for you! Even if you've had pain for years doesn't mean you are stuck suffering for the rest of your life.

The way doctors communicate with life sufferers is especially important. Just telling a patient that she has some wear and tear on her spine rather using than the scary term *arthritis* really helps the Life-Sufferer.

The Life-Sentence Sufferer can also be a quiet sufferer, chronic sufferer, or an acute sufferer. Anyone who does not seek treatment for his or her discomfort and thus lives with it, day in and day out, fits in this category. My hope is to give Life-Sentence sufferers their lives back. I have treated many people with these diagnoses and ongoing pain who now have *absolutely no pain.*

## 5. THE TRAUMATIC BACK SUFFERER

**"That accident really messed me up and there is nothing else that can be done."**

*Answer "yes" or "no" to the following statements to determine if you are a Traumatic Back Sufferer:*

|  | YES | NO |
|---|---|---|
| You have been involved in a motor vehicle accident. | ☐ | ☐ |
| You got hurt while playing sports. | ☐ | ☐ |
| You back pain came about after a slip or fall. | ☐ | ☐ |

*Get one "yes"? This is you!*

The only thing random in the body is trauma. A bad ski accident, a car crash, a rough tackle during a football game are all examples of trauma-induced pain. If you have suffered trauma, your back problem is unique; no two accidents are ever quite the same. The first step is to make sure that you have not done any significant damage. While I always like to consider the least invasive options first, surgery may be necessary for these injuries. The less-invasive treatments, however, also need to be utilized as you heal and recover, and therefore you still need to take many of the same steps as the other back pain sufferers.

It is paramount for Traumatic Sufferers to make sure that they have balance in all areas of the body. People who may have physically healed but didn't extinguish their digestive inflammation or emotional stress won't heal properly.

As I discussed, identifying the type of sufferer you are provides insight into your lifestyle and the way you cope with both physical and emotional issues. This is essential in determining the correct cause of your pain and then properly utilizing this book to arrive at your personalized solution.

Most doctors are concerned with the specific part of the body that hurts, and they don't pay attention to what the rest of your body is telling them. A single-approach structural solution may apply if you are a Life-Sentence Sufferer or a Traumatic Back Sufferer, but for the other types of pain sufferers, relief often lies in a combination solution. Even Life-Sentence Sufferers and Traumatic Back Sufferers find significant improvement when treating other areas of the body that impact the back, so don't disregard the digestive and emotional sections! Remember, a complete, multi-faceted treatment is the best treatment!

As you read this book, you'll learn to listen to your body, identify all of your structural, emotional and digestive issues, and come to understand the truth about your back pain. My purpose is to give you hope and options. You may have thought that you did everything that you could to rid yourself of your back pain, but I am sure you most certainly haven't. At best, you've explored 33% of the potential solutions, likely only the structural ones—maybe not even, if you've only focused on the structure of the back. While I would never attempt to tell you that I have helped everyone, my three-pronged approach has provided relief and helped people who fall into each of these categories, and you will read their stories later in the book. Remember, the three-week rule applies to even those who have been suffering for most of their lives. All types of back pain sufferers deserve a chance to feel better!

# Five reasons why your back pain treatments are failing!

It can be one of the most frustrating feelings to seek ongoing treatment for back pain, only to find that after much time and effort . . . you still have back pain. As with almost everything in life, what works for one person is not necessarily going to work for anyone else. However, in my years of practice, I have seen many people come in after treatments with other doctors that yielded no results. Here are five of the most common reasons that your back pain treatments might be failing.

### 1. You're in the wrong place at the wrong time

Unfortunately, when it comes to treatments for back pain, what you get is based on who you see. For instance, if you see a physical therapist, he or she will prescribe stretches and specific exercises, but if you see an orthopedist, he or she will likely prescribe anti-inflammatory medications and potentially surgery. For a treatment to be successful, you have to be in the right place at the right time with the right health care specialist.

You greatly increase your chances of being in the right place at the right time with the right person by doing The Back Pain Inflammation Index, figuring out where your pain is coming from and following my recommendations of what type of doctor or practitioner to see. From there, do your research! Ask around and get recommendations from your friends. Google potential doctors and see what you find out. Do they have ongoing projects in their field or were their last studies completed in 1963? By doing research and asking around, you are more likely to get treatments with which you feel confident with and that are effective.

### 2. You (and your doctor) assume the problem is where the pain is

If you or your doctor think that treating only the area where you are experiencing pain is the answer, think again! This method of treatment is not encompassing the big picture, and that means that you will be missing results.

Most doctors and patients expect that their back pain is indicative of a problem in the back. For most sufferers, the problem is not your back. When analyzing a back pain sufferer, it is always important to keep in mind that everything in your body is related. For instance, a foot imbalance could cause low back problems or a jaw imbalance could result in shoulder pain. If your doctor insists on looking at your body as separate regions, rather than an entire system of pieces that are all integrated and working together, find a new doctor. Regional exams broken up by neck, mid-back, and low back are doomed to fail—and that means frustration, wasted money, and ongoing pain.

### 3. Your doctor created your treatment plan based on an MRI result

Magnetic resonance imaging (MRI) has proven to be worthless when it comes to back pain—at least when an entire treatment plan is based solely on MRI results. That's because this type of imagery is insufficient to determine the cause of most back pain. While an MRI can help determine injury to ligaments and tendons, usually, the source of the pain is not where you feel it. This makes the MRI basically ineffective in creating a treatment plan for pain caused by something else.

### 4. Your doctor isn't looking at ALL of the three potential causes of back pain

That's right. There are THREE causes of back pain. Back pain is not just a muscular or a structural problem, but often a combination of structural imbalances, reactions to emotional stressors, and an improper diet. By only addressing one facet of cause, your doctor is missing 66% of the information (and 66% of your pain relief potential!)

### 5. Your diagnosis is a prescription of a lifetime of pain

Because our current system is solely based on the structural/anatomical model of treatment, our medical professionals have developed diagnoses designed to make them look intelligent, all the while convincing the back pain sufferers that they have a condition that will bother them for their whole life. Diagnoses such as degenerative disc disease, disc bulge, disc herniation, spinal stenosis, and arthritis are believed to be recipes for a lifetime of suffering or at the least a "bad back." In fact, this could not be farther from the truth! This book will help you identify your type of suffering, create a 100% solution, and eliminate your back pain—in just a few short weeks!

# 2

# UNDERSTANDING PAIN AND INFLAMMATION

Before we can get rid of our pain, we need to understand what it really is. Why? Well, getting rid of pain without understanding it is analogous to removing the battery from your smoke alarm because the noise is too loud. Pain is your body's attempt to tell you that something is wrong. It is your built-in warning device. While pain-killing drugs (when properly used) are one of the greatest advances in the history of medicine, unfortunately, these drugs—both prescribed and over-the-counter—are not being properly used. We are continually putting the body's warning system of pain on mute with medication instead of properly extinguishing the fire.

Back pain sufferers are among the vast number of people who misuse and therefore become pain-medication abusers and addicts. That's why my solution, The Sinett Solution, helps you get to the source of your pain and offers natural, medication-free strategies to free you from pain. The definition of health is a state of optimal function, not merely the absence of pain. My goal is for you the back pain sufferer to strive for this optimal function.

## THE UNDERLYING CAUSE OF BACK PAIN

Inflammation or swelling as well as redness and pain are normally part of a healthy immune response initiated to help your body protect an injured part and begin healing by producing elevated levels of cortisol to maintain the connective tissue. However, when your cortisol levels have been elevated for a prolonged period of time, you develop chronic inflammation, which actually destroys healthy tissue and has been found to cause cancer, diabetes, depression, heart disease, stroke, and Alzheimer's disease. I would add back pain—as well as tension in the muscles, ligaments, tendons, and discs—to this list. Chronic inflammation is what makes our backs susceptible to "going out" after we make simple movements.

There are three causes of inflammation resulting in back pain:

1. Structural inflammation
2. Nutritional or digestive inflammation
3. Emotional inflammation

Back pain is just the symptom of an inflammatory problem, but not recognizing this is the reason why so many people are needlessly suffering from back pain. The keys to ridding back pain are the same keys to ridding the body's inflammatory factor.

When examining a back pain sufferer, I am not looking for a blown-out disc or a pinched sciatic nerve. What I am looking for is a patient's overall inflammatory score. In this section, you will take the Inflammatory Back Pain test. The higher your score on the Back Pain Inflammation Index, the greater the chance that you will suffer from back pain and poor health.

The Back Pain Inflammation Index will tell you your overall inflammatory score, where your inflammation is coming from (remember, the problem may not be in your back!), how to reduce it through a specific self-treatment plan, and even which health professionals to seek out should you need additional care.

Eliminating as many inflammatory factors as possible is the prescription not only for having a back pain-free life but for a happy and healthier one as well. Back pain could be the greatest gift if it forces you to make healthy life changes. These changes could include a new exercise regimen, adjusting eating habits, or ending unhealthy relationships. My patient, Ollie is truly one of the most inspiring people that I know. She came to me with a myriad of symptoms and has truly embraced the three prongs to health. Her story reveals just how important it is to be attentive to your overall inflammatory score, and not just isolate one part of the triad.

• • •

I HADN'T BEEN *feeling well when I first went to Dr. Sinett. Medically, I had been checked out and everything was fine, but I felt lethargic, achy, stressed beyond belief, and had awful neck, shoulder, and foot pain. I was extremely unhappy with the quality of my life, but I didn't know where to begin.*

*Dr. Sinett was my angel. In a very non-threatening or preachy way, he explained to me that my issues were all fixable and that there was not one cause per se but rather a combination of physical, emotional, and nutritional forces that were causing me to feel like this. Though I politely listened to everything that was said during my initial visits, I mentally dismissed that emotions could be a driving force in the way I felt physically. The funny part was that I knew what he was saying was true, but I did not think it applied to me. Can we say "denial"?*

*But I had reached the bottom of the barrel so to speak—I don't think I could have sunk any lower. I was highly frustrated with myself and my life. It was out of this deep dissatisfaction that I found my motivation. I decided to really adopt Dr. Sinett's Three-Pronged Approach and made a commitment to be successful. I did not specifically write down any goals, but I knew in my head and heart what outcomes I wanted. Here are how I worked on my Three Prongs:*

EMOTIONAL

*If I had to identify one pivotal element in transforming my life, I have to give tremendous credit to Michael Lodish, a stress management and biofeedback counselor at Midtown Integrative Health and Wellness (Dr. Sinett's office), for helping me navigate the emotional cross currents of my life. I came to learn that my emotional health was a key driver of my physical and nutritional wellness. I openly shared with Mike areas of my life that I felt needed fixing or challenges I was facing. Together we mapped out a plan for tackling these items. To achieve success in emotional healing, I feel you really have to be committed, honest with yourself, and prepared to go outside of your comfort zone—none of which are easy by any means.*

*Tackling self-esteem issues were the most challenging. In working with Mike, I realized that I, not anyone or anything, was standing in the way of my own happiness. All the excuses I had been making for years were just a cover for fears that I had. Once everything was out in the open, I felt as if a great big weight had been lifted from my shoulders. In the months that followed, I felt more confident and became more social, really putting myself out there (something the old me would have never done). While it did not always manifest the way I had hoped, I learned a lot about myself in the process.*

*Work stressors were the easiest, relatively speaking. Mike's guidance was invaluable and provided the reinforcement I needed when doubt and insecurity would set in. I used to have to travel a few days per week out of state for work and have since made adjustments to my schedule so that I no longer feel like I don't have any time for myself. Additionally, I have applied more flexibility to my work hours to maintain better balance in my life.*

## STRUCTURAL

*I had started working out more regularly a few months before I came to see Dr. Sinett, but seeing him regularly motivated me to keep at it, especially as I often got discouraged. The combination of chiropractic adjustments and therapy helped me to keep limber, out of pain, and free of circulatory blocks. Two years ago, I couldn't even run two laps around the track. By last November, I participated in a local 5K Turkey Trot and most recently, I ran in the NYC Half Marathon. I only made it to Mile 11, but that's made me even more motivated to continue to train so I can try again next year and have greater success.*

## NUTRITIONAL

*During this time I gave up sugar (candies, cookies, cake, etc.), which was extremely tough for me, as I have been addicted to it my whole life. I wasn't the type of person who could just have one cookie . . . I could never have enough and the more I had it, the more I wanted. I have now learned to enjoy fruit. I limit the amount of carbs I eat and make healthier food choices overall. I found that by improving my emotional well-being, the need to lean on food for comfort has been drastically reduced. A byproduct of not eating sugar has been that my joints don't hurt like they used to!*

*I went on a rollercoaster ride of emotional ups and downs during all of this time of self-help. As I was getting closer to achieving personal success, there were times when self-doubt would creep in or I would allow negative thinking to take over or I would look to food for comfort. I had spent so much of my life comfortably buried under all the reasons why I couldn't be happy that when happiness was within sight, I was overcome with fear of actually experiencing it and would revert to what I knew best. You were able to recognize this and keep me from sabotaging myself.*

*I'm incredibly proud of how I feel today: happy. It's as if I'm standing on a mountaintop looking over the long path that I've walked to get here and taking stock of all the challenges, pain, hard work, and terrific people who helped me get to where I am. Overall my outlook on life (and the challenges that may present themselves, whether personal or professional) is very different today than a year ago. I feel happy, balanced, alive, confident, loved, valued, and complete. I am viewing life through a new set of lenses!*

*Olivera Radakovic*

## BACK PAIN DANGER SIGNS

Back pain can be a mild annoyance, or it can actually be a symptom of a serious medical condition. There are too many stories of people who have ignored their pain and symptoms only to realize that they were caused by an underlying disease. If you have any additional symptoms, such as serious back pain that wakes you up at night, back pain with fever, if you are unable to lift your foot while walking, if your back pain is accompanied by an inability to control your bowel or bladder function, numbness or tingling, or even severe back pain that has lasted more than two weeks, please seek help from a doctor who can examine you in person. If the following questions in the Back Pain Inflammation Index generally cover your array of symptoms and other issues you may be experiencing, proceed to calculate your total inflammatory score!

# THE BACK PAIN INFLAMMATION INDEX

The Back Pain Inflammation Index is the central diagnostic tool for The Sinett Solution. It is made up of the questions I ask my patients who come into the office in order to determine the correct source or sources of their pain, and this is what will help you arrive at the proper self-diagnosis and ultimately, the proper prescription. Now that you know the importance and the repercussions of inflammation, you understand why it is so important to answer these questions honestly and accurately! Remember, there is no shame in admitting you have been eating poorly or are in a tough spot in life. Honesty here will help you reduce all of the body's inflammation and help you find relief in three weeks.

The Back Pain Inflammation Index is broken down into three parts: structural questions, digestive questions, and emotional questions. Even if you think your problem is stemming from just one area, you must answer the questions in each of the three sections. Most of my patients don't connect all of their habits and behaviors to the back, and you will only arrive at the correct treatment if you address 100% of your body's needs. The Sinett Solution is about bringing all three systems of the body into balance, and many people do need to improve all of these areas in order to achieve optimum function and well-being.

To use the Index, give 0 points for each answer of "no" and 1 point for each "yes." You'll add up each section individually to determine how much inflammation is stemming from structural issues, how much is being caused by digestive upsets, and when emotional sources are leading to pain. You'll also add up all three numbers to determine your overall inflammatory score out of 100. These scores will help you diagnose yourself and will direct you to the correct sections of the book, so that you can form the right treatment plan.

## HOW MUCH IS STRUCTURAL?

Remember here that the only thing random in the body is trauma. If you fell off your bike and now your back hurts, that is trauma-induced pain. Otherwise, pain due to a structural cause is not random, and it doesn't occur from simply bending down incorrectly. This type of structural pain tends to be caused by a buildup of bad habits, such as sitting at your desk all day, or prolonged misuse of your body, which can develop in someone who has poor posture.

Answer the following questions to determine how much of your back pain is caused by structural issues. Remember, rate each question with a 0 for "no" and a 1 for "yes."

| | NO [0] | YES [1] |
|---|---|---|
| Did you recently exercise differently? | _____ | _____ |
| Did you recently lift anything heavier than normal? | _____ | _____ |
| Do you do sit-ups or crunches? | _____ | _____ |
| Do you sit at a computer for more than four hours a day? | _____ | _____ |
| Have you been traveling a lot? | _____ | _____ |
| Were you doing different types of work, such as shoveling snow or raking leaves? | _____ | _____ |
| Were you bent over in an unusual posture for a long period of time? | _____ | _____ |
| Have you been wearing different shoes? | _____ | _____ |
| Does your jaw click when talking or chewing? | _____ | _____ |
| Do you have difficulty placing at least three fingers in your mouth horizontally at one time? | _____ | _____ |
| Are your teeth, mouth, or gums sore when you wake up? | _____ | _____ |
| Do you get pain on the side of your head above your ear or elsewhere around the ear? | _____ | _____ |
| Do you feel as if you have frequent sinus infections? | _____ | _____ |
| Are you aware that you clench your teeth? | _____ | _____ |
| Has your dentist ever noted that you grind your teeth? | _____ | _____ |
| **TOTAL:** | | **YES** |

| | NO [0] | YES [1] |
|---|---|---|
| Do you suffer from headaches more than once every two weeks? | _____ | _____ |
| Can you turn your head further with your mouth open than with it closed? | _____ | _____ |
| Can you see or turn your head further with your arm raised above your head than with your arm down? | _____ | _____ |
| Do you tend to snore? | _____ | _____ |
| Do you have difficulty chewing? | _____ | _____ |
| Do you need to chew on one side of your mouth? | _____ | _____ |
| Do you get ear pain or feel the need to clear your ears when going up in elevation or when flying? | _____ | _____ |
| Do you read in bed? | _____ | _____ |
| Do you feel better with a pillow behind your back? | _____ | _____ |
| Do your neck and shoulders frequently feel tight? | _____ | _____ |
| Do you feel the need to twist or crack your own neck? | _____ | _____ |
| Do you feel the need for frequent massages? | _____ | _____ |
| Do you feel the need to hang on a bar or stretch upside-down? | _____ | _____ |
| Do your shoulders frequently bother you? | _____ | _____ |
| Do you ever get numbness or tingling in your arms, fingers, or wrists? | _____ | _____ |
| Do you have difficulty walking on your tippy toes? | _____ | _____ |
| Do you have difficulty walking on your heels? | _____ | _____ |
| Do your arms or hands frequently fall asleep? | _____ | _____ |
| Do you feel the need to be careful when you bend or lift? | _____ | _____ |

TOTAL: _____
                    YES

| | NO [0] | YES [1] |
|---|---|---|
| Have you had a severe back episode in the past two years? | _____ | _____ |
| Do you always need to be careful with your back? | _____ | _____ |
| Does sitting in the car aggravate your back? | _____ | _____ |
| Do you need to always find the perfect chair? | _____ | _____ |
| Have you noticed one hip being higher than the other? | _____ | _____ |
| Has your tailor noted that one side of your pants needs to be slightly longer? | _____ | _____ |
| Do your feet bother you? | _____ | _____ |
| Does your back bother you after standing? | _____ | _____ |
| Do your shoes or sneakers wear down differently? | _____ | _____ |
| Does your back feel better or worse depending on what shoes you wear? | _____ | _____ |
| Do your legs feel heavy? | _____ | _____ |
| Do your knees feel weak after standing or walking? | _____ | _____ |
| Is your computer monitor off to the side from where you are sitting? | _____ | _____ |
| Do you look down while texting or emailing? | _____ | _____ |
| Are you in the car for more than seven hours a week? | _____ | _____ |
| Have you ever bent down and had trouble standing back up? | _____ | _____ |

TOTAL: _____
YES

*Add up your total score for this section.*

GRAND TOTAL: _____
YES

**5 POINTS OR LESS**

If you have 5 or fewer points, chances are the problem is not structural, but rather stems from a digestive or emotional issue.

**5-10 POINTS**

If your total is between 5 and 10 points, you are at moderate risk for back pain due to structural causes. Reading the structural solutions section will help you identify where your structural aggravations are coming from and integrate better habits into your daily life to nip your pain in the bud! The Backbridge™ will be the answer for many in this category!

**10+ POINTS**

If your score is 10 or more points, you must get to work now! You have been in too much pain and need to feel better. Your solution may also require digestive and emotional elements, but you certainly have structural imbalances that, once corrected, will enable you to find relief. Go to Section 1: Structural Solutions to find the particular root of your pain and what to do to fix it.

# HOW MUCH IS DIGESTIVE?

What you eat—whether it's too much coffee, too many sweets or a host of other edibles—can agitate your digestive system and chemically induce back pain. Even the healthiest of eaters can suffer digestive-related back pain! With dietary issues, we are looking for either changes in the chemical system or repetitive patterns that can result in back pain. Hormonal changes also fall into the Digestive/Chemical category and can profoundly influence back health. These questions will help you assess your digestive and hormonal inflammatory factor. Answer yes or no to each question, giving 1 point for yes and 0 points for a no.

|  | NO [0] | YES [1] |
|---|---|---|
| Have you been constipated recently? | ____ | ____ |
| Have you had diarrhea recently? | ____ | ____ |
| Has your stomach been bothering you? | ____ | ____ |
| **TOTAL:** | | **YES** |

|  | NO [0] | YES [1] |
|---|---|---|
| Have you had an increase in gas? | _____ | _____ |
| Have you eaten any types of food that you don't normally consume? | _____ | _____ |
| Have you eaten spicy foods recently? | _____ | _____ |
| Have you recently had a stomach virus? | _____ | _____ |
| Have you been on any new medications? | _____ | _____ |
| Have you changed your diet? | _____ | _____ |
| Have you changed your vitamin regimen? | _____ | _____ |
| Have you increased your fiber intake? | _____ | _____ |
| Do you tend to have the same meals more than three times in a week? | _____ | _____ |
| Do you eat five large raw salads or more in a week? | _____ | _____ |
| Have you recently started to drink five or more fruit smoothies in a week? | _____ | _____ |
| Are you taking more than three different vitamins in a day? | _____ | _____ |
| Have you recently become a vegetarian? | _____ | _____ |
| Do you eat five or more cups of fruits and vegetables in a day? | _____ | _____ |
| Have you recently started to drink something different? | _____ | _____ |
| Have you drunk more than four alcoholic beverages in one sitting in the past week? | _____ | _____ |
| Do you depend on coffee or soda to stay awake during the day? | _____ | _____ |
| Do you have coffee at least once a day? | _____ | _____ |

TOTAL:                                    YES

|  | NO [0] | YES [1] |
|---|---|---|
| Do you use protein bars as meal replacements? | _____ | _____ |
| Do you eat more than one small dessert or treat during the day? | _____ | _____ |
| Do you use an artificial sweetener? | _____ | _____ |
| Do you have irregular bowel movements? | _____ | _____ |
| Have you been diagnosed with IBS (Irritable Bowel Syndrome)? | _____ | _____ |
| Do you turn to food when you're stressed or upset? | _____ | _____ |
| Do you skip meals? | _____ | _____ |
| Do you ever eat when you're not hungry or continue eating after you're full? | _____ | _____ |
| Do you eat at your desk? | _____ | _____ |
| Did you just begin your menstrual period or have you recently started menopause? | _____ | _____ |
| Has your hormonal system undergone any recent changes (menopause, change in birth control, missed menstrual period, pregnancy, etc.)? | _____ | _____ |

**TOTAL:**                   **YES** _____

*Add up your total score for this section.*

**GRAND TOTAL:**                   **YES** _____

### 4 POINTS OR LESS
If you have 4 points or less, you are at low risk for a digestive cause of back pain. Your cause is likely structural and/or emotional.

### 5-10 POINTS
If you total between 5 and 10 points, you are at moderate risk, which means digestive issues are probably a contributing factor to your back pain. You could find some relief by trying my No More Back Pain Diet and

identifying and eliminating foods that are particularly irritating to you to reduce your internal inflammation.

### 10+ POINTS

If you score more than 10 points, your back pain has a digestive root. Use Section 2: Digestive Solutions to begin your digestive evaluation and find the right nutrition plan to help reduce your stomach and back pain.

## HOW MUCH IS EMOTIONAL?

Stress causes tight muscles, and tight muscles can cause serious pain. Although many people are often reluctant to admit there is an emotional cause for their back pain, it is very important that you be open-minded about this cause, as we find that stress is a major contributor to back pain. (You'll read more about this later in the book.) Answer these questions using the same point system in the previous section.

| | NO [0] | YES [1] |
|---|---|---|
| Would you describe your current stress level as moderate to high? | ____ | ____ |
| Are you under particular stress at work? | ____ | ____ |
| Are you getting along with your fellow employees? | ____ | ____ |
| Do you feel better during the weekend compared to during the week? | ____ | ____ |
| Are you unemployed? | ____ | ____ |
| Are you concerned that you will be unemployed in the near future? | ____ | ____ |
| Have you recently had any financial problems? | ____ | ____ |
| Are you feeling fulfilled in your career? | ____ | ____ |
| Has there recently been a change in your relationships with your family members and friends? | ____ | ____ |
| **TOTAL:** | | **YES** |

|  | NO [0] | YES [1] |
|---|---|---|

Has a close family member or friend recently undergone an illness or a death? _____ _____

Did you recently have to do something that you didn't want to do? _____ _____

Do you frequently feel anxious? _____ _____

Do you seem to carry your stress in your upper body? More specifically, have you had headaches, tight neck, shoulder tension, or lower back pain? _____ _____

Are you trying to get pregnant but having difficulty doing so? _____ _____

Are you having trouble sleeping? _____ _____

Are you feeling stressed out and worried because of the pain you are suffering? _____ _____

Is anything else in your life happening that makes you feel stressed? _____ _____

TOTAL:          YES

*Add up your total score for this section.*

GRAND TOTAL:          YES

### 3 POINTS OR LESS

If you have three or fewer points, you have excellent stress management skills, and your back pain probably doesn't have an emotional source.

### 4-6 POINTS

If you get between 4 and 6 points, stress is a moderate contributor to your back pain. When things get you tense, your back tightens up, and while it may not last forever, it does impact your comfort level from time to time, and is probably a recurring issue. Adopting some of my Enerchi balancing or other relaxation techniques will help you change your stress response and keep your emotionally induced back pain at bay.

**6 OR MORE POINTS**

If you score more than 6 points, your back pain is definitely stemming from your emotions, and you need to make serious changes in your stress reactions. My Three Week Enerchi Balancing Plan in Section 3 will offer ways to heal yourself from the inside out and will help you change your coping mechanisms. Doing so will allow you to control your stress and stay healthy—for good.

| SECTION | SCORE |
|---------|-------|
| Structural | |
| Digestive | |
| Emotional | |
| Total | |

This total number gives you a bird's eye view of the state of your back and overall health. The higher the total number, the more work you will have to do—and likely in all three areas of treatment. Remember, back problems are usually multi-faceted and by not addressing ALL of these factors, the core solution is lost. Likely, you'll see you have some points coming from each section. The highest number will tell you the most significant cause of your pain, but that doesn't mean you should ignore the lower numbers. These are places that need work, too. Without this inter-relationship approach, success is just about impossible. If you only treat one aspect of the triad, back pain will always lurk around. That is why we have so many quiet managers!

My patient, Maria, is just one example of a quiet manager who finally succumbed to a major backache after ignoring structural and emotional issues!

•   •   •

PRIOR TO VISITING *Dr. Sinett, I had a very hectic lifestyle with two young children, a very demanding job as a concierge, and a long commute every day. I had been having back issues for quite a while and had just been "dealing with it," which is not the best approach for back or personal care!*

*One day, my back went out, and I was not able to move. I had visited Dr. Sinett's father before his passing and I knew of their practice, but only knew Dr. Todd Sinett as "the son."*

*I didn't know much about kinesiology, and I was skeptical at first. But Todd's magical touch made all the difference. I saw him three times a week and was given both kinesiology treatments as well as adjustments, paired with heat and stimulation. He gave me a detailed plan of what I had to do to achieve a good back. It was a very holistic approach for your body, mind, and spirit. He was able to open my chi and realign the flow. He also helped me put things into perspective; his calm, common-sense approach to my issues made me see things as they really were, not as I thought they were in my head.*

*Dr. Sinett has changed my life in SOOOO many ways. He loves small catch phrases, like "Fake it till you make it," or "What you perceive you receive." So I live by those and many more of his smart common sense comments. He taught me the word CONGRUENT. And he could tell just by looking at me and my energy and the way I carried my body if I was being congruent.*

*The moment I will never forget is when Dr. Sinett said, "Maria, you have graduated!" He knew I had "figured it out." Now, when I do those things that are "un-congruent," such as get no sleep, find myself in an unhealthy relationships, take on too much, etcetera, Dr. Sinett has given me the tools and tips to handle my stress and everyday hardships myself. He has helped me remember, no matter what happens in life, to stay positive and not take yourself so darn seriously.*

*For me the most important part is to continue the treatment, to be proactive, and realize that seeing your chiropractor is a sure way of staying healthy and happy . . . and pain-free! I have sent so many guests, friends, and colleagues to Dr. Sinett, and they all felt like they had met the miracle maker and healer that Dr. Sinett has always been to me!*

*Maria Wittorp-Dejonge*

## Commit to 21 days!

By taking the BPI test, you have figured out where your pain is coming from and you will next learn how to formulate your specific action steps. In order to have success, you must commit to three weeks of self-treatment—in every area that needs work. Half-hearted efforts lead to half-hearted results. Maria gave herself the chance to find relief. Give yourself the 21-day shot at a pain-free life!

# The MRI Myth

Lots of doctors—and thus their patients—still believe that an MRI, or magnetic resonance imaging, is helpful in diagnosing back pain. In fact, this testing is so common that many of my patients come in and demand that I send them for an MRI. They think the pain must be the result of a disc or bone pressing on a nerve root and believe the MRI can be used to observe what is happening to the nerve. Stanley J. Bigos, professor emeritus of orthopedic surgery and environmental health at the University of Washington, explained the appeal of the MRI when he said, "The reality is patients want an answer, the doctor wants to get the patient out of the room and the hypotheses start to flow."

For some reason, the studies done that refute the power of the MRI have not resonated. For example, a study published in the *New England Journal of Medicine* in 1994 reported that MRIs were conducted on 98 people who were symptom-free of back pain. Sixty-four percent of these people showed clear evidence of a bulging or protruding disc and 28 percent showed disc herniation—spinal abnormalities that would seem to indicate severe back ailments. But because these people did not complain of back pain, the idea of diagnosing pain solely from an MRI is misguided.

Doctors at the University of Washington in Seattle then concluded in 1998 and 2000 that MRIs resulted in a higher rate of specialist consultations and more surgeries but *fewer* beneficial outcomes. In 2003, the *Journal of the American Medical Association* detailed a controlled randomized trial which proved that X rays were better than MRIs for diagnosing issues of lower back pain and resulted in fewer patient interventions and ultimately fewer surgeries.

Why don't MRIs produce better outcomes for back pain sufferers? It is because MRIs do not take the root cause into account. They serve only to bolster the notion that back pain is nothing more than the symptom of an underlying disease. Many conventional physicians and surgeons miss the true causes of back pain because they continue to focus on the easy explanation offered by high-tech imaging. All too often, the orthopedist who sees a herniated disc on an MRI decides that the only answer is surgery.

When no structural abnormality is found, patients are typically sent off with a prescription for anti-inflammatory drugs or other pain-killers. Pain-killers are not real solutions. They are not a cure. They merely mask the pain.

Because you now understand that the body is interconnected, you can see how finding and fixing even a localized issue means that both the doctor and the patient are missing the bigger picture—including a number of potential causes of your pain. If your back pain is caused by a foot imbalance, an MRI of the back will not tell you this. If your back pain is caused by emotional stress or a digestive upset, an MRI won't tell you this either! Localized issues can be improved—without surgery—by fixing the global issues.

So, when it comes to back pain, what are MRIs good for? They are helpful in diagnosing infection, fractures, and tumors, and they are great at telling what you don't have, as opposed to what you do have. But, ultimately, "true but unrelated" sums up MRI findings. They may find structural irregularities, causing the doctor to attempt to connect your symptoms to those irregularities. It's time to renounce these unreliable findings! My model, which takes into account all of the possible sources of global pain, will tell you so much more about your body and why you are suffering than an MRI ever could. And with that core information can come an effective (and less invasive) solution—the Sinett Solution!

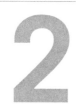
# Structural Causes and Solutions

# 3

# SEARCHING FOR
# THE STRUCTURAL CAUSES

## THE PAIN MAY NOT BE WHERE THE PROBLEM IS!

f you have been directed to this section, your structural inflammation score was moderate to high, and your pain is caused, at least in part, by structural issues, or something wrong in the bones, muscles, or nerves, most often generated by habits and posture that are not "structurally sound."

As you move forward with your structural diagnosis, you should note that back pain is really spine pain. All nerves exit the spine so improving the function of the spine can have a profound impact on your entire body. I still receive bewildered looks when a patient's knee or wrist pain is reduced by treating his or her back. When you expand your knowledge and understanding of your spine and realize the impact a balance or imbalance can have on various parts of the body, you will grasp a very important concept in structural treatment. Back pain can refer to and include most any type of pain.

You see, there are two types of structural back problems:

1. Localized Issues, or conditions that our medical model seems to approach properly because the problem is actually at the site of the pain. A localized herniated disc or a specific injury will respond to the traditional care from the necessary specialist (a physical therapist, orthopedist, etc.). For a muscular issue, manual therapy combined with some stretches usually does the trick.

2. Compensatory/global issues. Most causes of back pain are not local problems but rather a global spinal reaction. While a patient may be complaining of a particular symptom or pain, there is usually a much wider area of involvement.

To understand this concept, visualize your spine as a shoelace. Take that shoelace and staple one end of the lace to a piece of paper and let the other end hang down. This is your spine. Now start twisting the loose end of the shoelace. If you twist long enough, you'll find that the entire shoelace—as well as the piece of paper (which represents the rest of your body)—gets all twisted. Now you understand that what happens in one location in your spine most definitely affects the rest of your body. The spine is completely integrated and relates to your entire body. If you view your body as a compilation of separate and distinct parts, the likelihood of ridding yourself of back pain forever is nearly impossible. As you begin to understand your structural diagnosis, keep in mind that the body is interconnected and your treatment may target a spot where you don't particularly feel the pain.

• • •

As a professional tennis player and teacher from Mali, Africa, I had been suffering from severe groin pains. Playing tennis was unthinkable—just standing and feeding tennis balls during my lessons was downright painful! To get through the day, I had to take tons of anti-inflammatories, even though the medication was really messing up my stomach. I had been to the best doctors in New York City and they told me to rest, ice, and take the anti-inflammatories, but after three months, it was only getting worse.

When I gave Dr. Todd Sinett a tennis lesson, I never thought that my life would change forever. Dr. Sinett saw how I was limping and wearing this enormous ace bandage and he asked about my problem. I told him about my severe groin pain and how long it had been going on. He was kind enough to offer to examine me at his office to see if he could help me. I certainly didn't think he could help but considering the options, why not? Once he examined me, Dr. Sinett explained that he didn't think the pain was a groin problem, but rather a problem coming from my foot. He adjusted my foot, and I immediately felt better. He did this two more times at follow-up appointments, and I was 100% cured. Since I *work on my feet all day, it made sense that an imbalance in my foot could radiate all the way up my leg and into my groin. Dr. Sinett has turned out to be a great friend and an inspiration. I have gone on to open my own tennis club and certainly could not have done this without feeling better. I am a living example of how the Sinett method changes lives for the better!*

*Moussa Drame*

## A QUICK ANATOMY LESSON FOR THE STRUCTURAL SUFFERER

The spine is a dynamic structure designed for both strength and flexibility. It has three major functions:

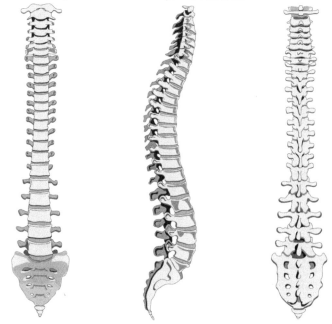

Figure 1. The anatomy of the spine.

1. To keep us upright
2. To protect the spinal cord, which carries our brain's messages to our outlying nerves. This is a fundamental component of our body's nervous system, the master computer for our bodies,

*(continued on next page)*

*(continued from previous page)*

which allows us to have good balance and react to our sur-
roundings, such as removing our hands from a hot surface.
3. To allow us to bend and move.

The spinal column consists of 33 vertebrae, 24 of which are
mobile and give the body and spine its flexibility. The vertebrae, both mobile and immobile, are linked, and they are
connected by joints called facets. These facets are separated
by discs, which are made of a jelly-like substance and provide
stability and cushioning to the spine.

Numerous muscles and ligaments are attached to the vertebrae. Each of these muscles performs certain actions that play an
integrated role in overall function. Imbalance in any one of these
muscles can throw off the intricate balance of any spine. Continued imbalance results in a decrease of function and often pain!

Compensatory/global imbalances are the most common sources of pain.
These imbalances come from five specific spinal "choke points," or places
in the body that affect not only the spine but the entire body. In addition to
being the most common, they are the easiest to fix. The problem is that they
are also the most overlooked, which explains why you've been suffering for
so long. Finding these global imbalances is the key to treatments that have
long-lasting impact. Just as in in building a house (you don't put the floors
down until the walls are up and painted), there is a natural order of healing
that must be followed. All global/compensatory imbalances must be corrected first before addressing a patient's localized problem. Once you have
removed the global/compensatory issues, the majority of patients feel significantly better, necessitating less work to be done on the localized issue.

Unfortunately, insurance companies only cover the examination and
treatment of the area where the patient is suffering and complaining
of pain, but when evaluating one's spine and back, a physician must
examine a patient from head to toe. If you have imbalance in any of
the five choke points, you will not be able to rid yourself of back pain.
Regional exams such as only examining a patient's lower back simply
won't work. The feet, the pelvis, the core/mid-thoracic region, the neck,
and the temporal mandibular joint are the five "choke points" that affect

the entire spine. Remember, the problem for most is not the back. The structural problems for most patients are actually occurring in one of these five choke points:

## CHOKE POINT #1: The Feet

The foot is constructed with three arches which, when properly maintained, give exceptional supportive strength. These three arches form a supporting vault that distributes the weight of the entire body.

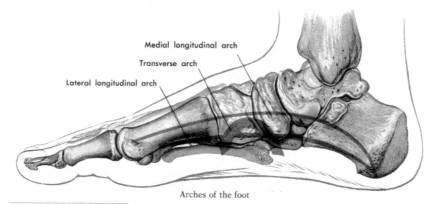

Medial longitudinal arch

Transverse arch

Lateral longitudinal arch

Arches of the foot

*Source: Posturepro*

But for many people who suffer from back pain, certain areas within their feet do not carry their end of the bargain, causing an imbalance that reverberates all the way up the spine.

The pen trick is a great way to demonstrate how a small imbalance in the foot can affect a seemingly unrelated body part. Choose a partner with good arm and shoulder function. Have him hold his arm out to the side and try to push his arm down with some mild to moderate pressure. The person should be able to hold his arm up against the resistance. Once you see that this person is able to do this, place a pen under one of his feet and have him stand on it. Retest the muscle strength. The strength should be dramatically reduced. While this sounds like hocus pocus, it will actually work on every single person. Why? It's based on normal neurology. There are messages that go from the brain throughout the body and messages that go from the body back to the brain for interpretation. These messages or impulses are called afferent and efferent impulses (don't worry, I won't get too technical). So what is happening when the foot is standing on the pen?

The foot sends the message to the brain that it is off-balance, and when the body is off-balance, the entire muscular system can't function optimally. These neurological impulses are the same reason why a pebble in your shoe becomes so painful or you know to pull your hand away from a hot stove. In the pen trick, the brain easily tells the foot to get off of the pen in order to re-center itself, but when there is a habitual, unconscious imbalance (caused by poor footwear, bad posture, or something else), the brain can't give a clear message, so it's up to you to tune in and fix the problem.

There are several ways to determine if you have an imbalance in your feet:

1. Look at the bottom of your shoes. Shoes should wear down evenly from left to right and both shoes should wear down the same way at the same rate. If this does not occur, you can safely assume that your feet are not in balance.
2. Pay attention to how you feel after wearing different types of shoes. If your footwear choices seem to affect how both your back or overall body feels, your feet could be the missing piece in ridding yourself of back pain. Remember to always listen to your body.
3. If you answered "yes" to any of these questions in the Back Pain Inflammatory Test:
   • Do your feet bother you?
   • Does your back bother you after standing?
   • Do your shoes or sneakers wear down differently?
   • Does your back feel better or worse depending on what shoes you wear?

Here's one patient's story about how she tuned into what her feet were telling her and consequently discovered a simple solution to her problem. The point of this story is to show you how interconnected your body is and also to give an example of how the body speaks a language.

●　●　●

MY FEET WERE CAUSING ME PAIN!

AT THE END *of a work day, I would literally feel as if I had no strength in my legs. My knees would ache, and my feet and my back would be sore. I could not wait to get home. I thought everyone felt this way after a day of standing on their feet, but Dr. Todd told me he was on his feet all day too and he felt fine. He suggested orthotics, or molded insoles. With orthotics in my shoes, I regained balance in my feet and all the strength returned to my legs, without any pain in my feet, back, or knees. This was a complete life changer for me.*

*Erin Weissman*

Today, appearance seems to take priority over function. Back pain caused by poor shoes is much more frequent during the warm summer months or in warmer climates because people tend to wear flip flops, open-toe shoes, and sandals. Women tend to suffer even more; heels that are higher than three inches put too much of your body weight on the front of the foot, which can cause calluses, bunions, corns, and hammertoes and strain your arches. Flats don't support your arch or Achilles tendon and if you wear them too frequently, can cause your foot to become pronated, or flattened. A laced up or strapped shoe always provides more support than an open back shoe.

> **TIP:** Be mindful of when your shoes feel like they are wearing down and replace them. Stretching out the life of a tired shoe only leads to added foot imbalance and back pain! When shopping, look for shoes that have room around the toes to prevent blisters, cushioning in the arch, the ball, and the heel, and a sole that is thickest at the back to provide slight elevation. Remember, a flip flop or shoes with an open back offer the least heel support!

Still, shoes are generally only designed for the mass public. A portion of the population won't function well in shoes made for the masses and will need a shoe designed and molded specifically for their unique feet. Orthotics work by customizing your sneakers, shoes and even high heels so that your foot sits properly in the shoe and is therefore able to strike properly. There are full and half orthotics. If you want to try an over-the-counter orthodic, the brand I like is Walkfit. They are significantly less expensive than a fully customized one. However, if you want to invest in a customized product, the orthodics I use are made by Footlevelers. The Footleveler orthotic is made by getting either a mold or a computerized foot scan of your weight distribution while standing. Footleveler designs the orthotic specifically for your feet, allowing you to evenly distribute your body's weight. Some chiropractors and podiatrists will make a mold of your feet. Professionally made orthotics can be costly, from $200 to $800, although some health insurers cover a portion of the cost. Just make sure there is a return policy in case they aren't a perfect fit!

## CHOKE POINT #2: The Pelvis

The pelvis is the lower most part of the spine. I describe the pelvis as the foundation of the house with the head, neck, and shoulders representing the second floor. Just imagine the far-reaching effects a crooked foundation can have. Within the pelvis are your hips. If your pelvis is not aligned properly, it can easily affect your hips and your entire lower extremity including your knees and legs. It is extremely rare to be born with one leg longer or shorter than the other. If your tailor tells you that you need one pant leg longer than the other, most likely you have pelvic imbalance!

Evaluating pelvic balance is easily accomplished by standing in front of the mirror and placing your hands on each side of your pelvis. Ideally, your hands should line up perfectly. The extent (in degrees) that a person's pelvis is off-balance can be measured by a lower back X ray. The larger the differential between each side of the pelvis, the greater the chances are that a patient is suffering from back pain.

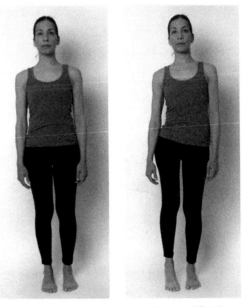

Balanced Pelvis    Imbalanced Pelvis

Pelvic imbalance can be caused by something simple, such as having your wallet in your back pocket and sitting on it all day. Even a tiny imbalance such as this is enough to tilt your pelvis and create reverberating back pain! Take a look at this man. You can see how the wallet in his back pocket bulges! Sitting on this causes one glute to be raised higher than the other:

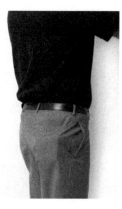

> **TIP:** Pelvis balancing solutions including laying over a big exercise ball, the Backbridge™, physical therapy or chiropractic adjustments, or using orthotics in your shoes. Even just taking your wallet out of your back pocket and making sure that your desk and chair are centered helps ensure that your pelvis is properly aligned.

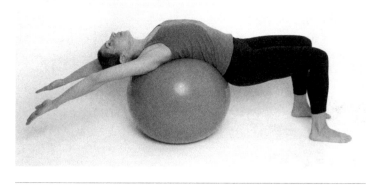

If structural treatments don't seem to work, there could be some other factors. The muscles that stabilize your pelvis relate to the adrenal glands, or your stress glands. When your body is under stress (either from emotional or nutritional causes), the pelvic stabilizing muscles become compromised, making pelvic balance impossible. The solutions may be to change your diet, reduce your sugar intake, and ease your overall stress.

## CHOKE POINT #3: The Core and Mid-Thoracic

Core/mid-thoracic imbalance is so prevalent that it is rare to find a person who doesn't suffer from it. This is because we spend the majority of our days hunched over a computer, and our bodies get an inordinate amount of forward bending, resulting in core imbalance and too much pressure in our mid-thoracic back. Our posture develops rounded shoulders, tight chest muscles, and forward movement of our head. This has become such a workplace epidemic that "sitting is the new smoking" has become the hot new catchphrase.

My patients feel the toll sitting is taking on their body and actually see it in the mirror in their posture. "I don't want to be a hunchback," they say, but they seem resigned to their fate. They can't quit their day job, after all!

The solution is learning how to engage the extensor muscles and disengage our flexor muscles to strike a balance between forward bending and back-bending.

I have developed the Backbridge™ to help put much needed extension back into our core and mid-thoracic zone. The Backbridge™ works by engaging the extensors while disengaging the overworked flexors. Pages 99-112 are devoted to the Backbridge™ (or an alternate option you may already have at home) and the ways it can ease your pain in just two minutes a day and change your life!

Other anti-flexion exercises that can help you find relief include: the cobra pose in yoga, the Thumbs to Pits stretch, or the Brugger's Relief Position.

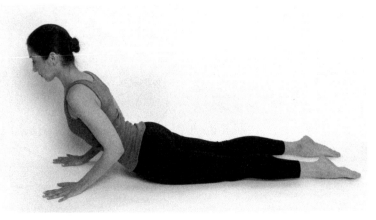

The cobra pose in yoga

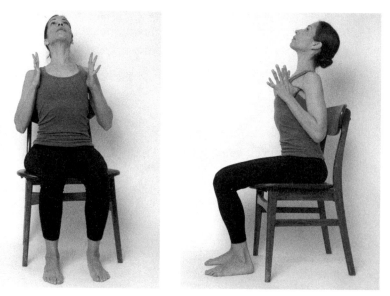

The Thumbs to Pits stretch

## BRUGGER'S RELIEF POSITION

**1.** Sit at the edge of a chair.

**2.** Place your feet directly below the knees and then separate them slightly and turn them slightly outward.

**3.** Roll the pelvis slightly forward to lightly arch the low back.

**4.** Ease the sternum forward and upward slightly.

**5.** Rotate your arms outward so your palms face forward.

**6.** Separate your fingers and point your thumbs backward.

**7.** Draw the chin in slightly.

**8.** Hold this position while taking a deep breath in through your abdomen.

**9.** Repeat several times per hour if you are sedentary.

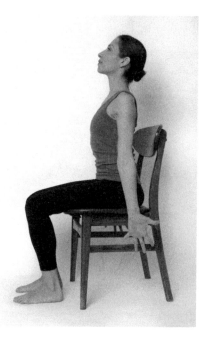

▶ **TIP:** Proper ergonomics can help anyone who spends their time desk-bound for long days. Here's what you should know about setting up a proper workstation:

- Your chair should maintain all of your spinal curves when sitting with good lower back support.
- The chair should be on wheels so that you can pull yourself into a comfortable position with feet resting lightly on the floor. If you are short, you may need a stool underneath your desk.
- The chair should also be able to extend back to allow you to stretch and relieve compression.
- Adjust your monitor so that your head is straight when looking at it.

### DON'T JUST SIT THERE

Essentially, sitting compresses the body, stacking one spinal disc on top of another. Our muscles, which are designed to move, are now resigned to a state of stagnant contraction! To help your muscles relax and stave off core/mid-thoracic imbalance:

- Shift your weight every few minutes. Arch your back, shift from side to side, or lean back to relieve the forward hunch.

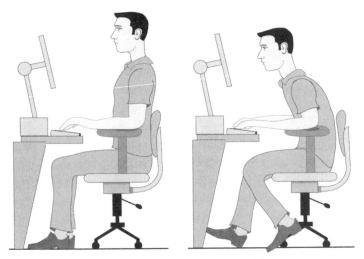

Correct vs. incorrect office chair position

- Stand up and shift your weight from one foot to the other. This is great to do while you are on the phone!
- Set the alarm on your phone or computer, and every 30 minutes, get up and walk around—grab supplies, change the printer paper, or refill your water bottle. Anything to get up and move for a minute!
- Do the standing abdominal stretch (see page 81).

### Sitting Pretty

Sitting is hard on the body and since you often don't have a choice in what type of chair you use, you should look into other solutions to help you maintain a healthy core. Here is my list of seats that are bad for us and the ways to maintain a healthy core/mid-thoracic while sitting in them:

**Stools**: Good posture and stools, whether at the bar or your kitchen counter, do not go hand in hand. Because most people curl over and lean on the bar or counter, stools reinforce the compression factor. Instead, sit up on the stool with your pelvis tipped forward slightly. The waist is not a hinge, so don't bend there. If your feet are suspended, rest them on a rail under the stool.

**Restaurant Booths**: If they are narrow enough to let you lean back or if they are firm enough that you can perch forward, sit, again, with your pelvis tilted forward and shoulders back. Ideally, restaurants with bench seating will provide pillows that you can place behind your back, allowing diners to "custom fit" their seat.

**Molded Seats**: These seats, found on buses and in some restaurants, are designed to crunch the pelvis toward the torso, which is not good for you! If you're forced to sit on one of these, perch forward and sit up straight.

**The Couch**: We all need somewhere cozy to curl up, but it is healthier for your spine if you prop the pillows behind you to create support for your back. A slight backward tilt is ideal!

If you are going to be sitting, find a chair that reclines back such as a La-Z-Boy. A reclined chair lengthens the spine, eliminating a good amount of the harmful effects of sitting.

## CHOKE POINT #4: The Neck

Most people forget to discuss the role the neck plays in back pain. The neck represents the top of the spine, which is intricately linked to the entire body. Nerves exiting the neck travel throughout the spine, so an imbalance within the neck can cause *both* upper and lower back pain. The neck's job is to support the weight of your head. A helpful analogy is that the head should sit on your neck like a golf ball would sit on a tee. Since your head weighs about the same as a bowling ball, the proper alignment and balance in your neck is really important. A neck and head not in alignment can easily lead to pain. If this goes on for a prolonged period of time you may get significant amount of pain. It is as if your head becomes too heavy for your neck to support!

Balance in the neck is also particularly important because the neck controls the messages that go to and from the brain and the majority of mechanoreceptors in the body. Mechanoreceptors essentially tell your body where you are in space, so a neck imbalance can cause dizziness and balance issues.

Neck pain can begin from a trauma such as a fall or a motor vehicle accident or just from day-to-day activities, such as sitting in front of a computer for hours at a time. One of the most frequent causes is what I call the dreaded "Shoulder Phone Clamp." Today, I have many more phone-pain patients than at the start of my career because everyone is now glued to their cell phone—and the phones keep getting smaller and smaller, which means we are crunching our neck more and more to keep the device steady between shoulder and ear. This simple move, when done repetitively, intensifies the tension in the neck and shoulder and robs you of flexibility in that area. Symptoms from neck tension can be headaches, numbness going down the arms, pain in the shoulder and shoulder blades, low back pain, and even wrist or elbow pain.

When treating the neck, I strive to help a patient achieve a normal range of motion and flexibility. For the most part, neck pain will improve with some cervical traction (stretching or lengthening the neck), physical therapy, massage, stretching, and chiropractic adjustments. It is important to make sure that the treatment is not too aggressive at the beginning and that you ease into the stretches. My online neck video will help you get started. Before you do the stretches, see how flexible your neck is and then retest it after you perform the stretches. This way you can evaluate how much benefit you received. Over time, these stretches should have a profound impact on your neck flexibility.

# NECK STRETCH SEQUENCE

This quick sequence give you a light neck stretch of lateral flexion in both directions, as well as flexion, extension, and rotation:

## 1. Lateral Flexion

Sitting up tall, gently bring your right ear to your right shoulder. Place your right hand over your left ear and gently guide your head toward the right shoulder. Hold for ten seconds. Repeat on the other side.

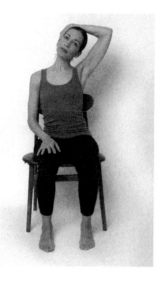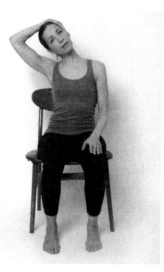

## 2. Flexion

Sitting up tall, bring your chin toward your chest, place your fingertips behind your head, and guide your head forward toward your chest. Hold for a count of ten.

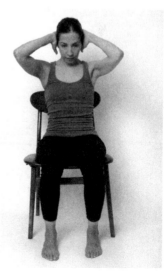

### 3. Extension

Now, bring your chin up. Gently place your hands on the back of your head and let your head fall further backward. Make sure that this stretch is comfortable and that you are not getting light-headed or dizzy. Hold for a count of ten and bring your head forward again.

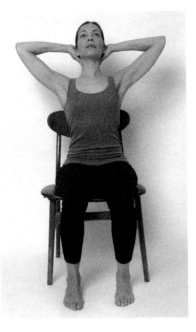

### 4. Rotation

Sitting up tall, turn your chin toward your right shoulder. Then place your right hand on the left side of the face and gently guide your head and chin to the right shoulder. Hold for ten seconds then repeat on other side.

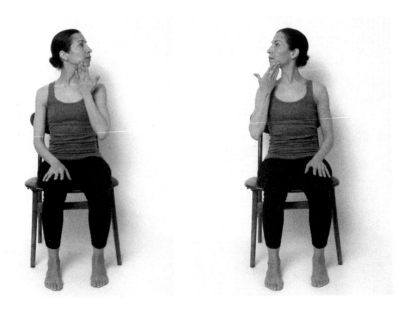

Other possible solutions include:

**Backbridge™.** A lot of neck pain comes from poor posture and forward rounded shoulders. The Backbridge™ restores much-needed extension into your back, helping that shoelace effect in the neck.

**Mouth guard.** TMJ dysfunction will frequently cause neck pain, so using a mouth guard when you're sleeping at night can help alleviate pain originating in the jaw that radiates down to the neck. They are available over the counter and custom molded.

**Try a proper pillow.** When sleeping, ideally you want your head to be lower than your neck so that the head and neck can completely relax. Some posture-pedic pillows have dips in the center to allow the neck to be held up in high support. The only problem with these pillows is that as you move around in the night, your neck and head don't always wind up in the correct position, rendering these pillows ineffective. The solution is a water pillow; the water will get displaced to properly support your neck and head, no matter which way you move! Chiroflow water pillows is my favorite brand, available at chiroflow.com.

**Investing in a headset.** Goodbye Shoulder Phone Clamp!

**Try your own TENS Unit.** For tight and stiff muscles in your upper back and shoulders as well as your lower back, try a TENS Unit. TENS Units are able to mimic the effects of electrotherapy to the muscles safely in your own home, helping to reduce pain and inflammation all throughout the body. The one I recommend is made by Trumedic.

▶ **TIP: HEADS UP!** Every inch or ten degrees that your neck is bent forward and down while texting or reading increases the weight or strain on your neck by 10 pounds. So if you are bent 60 degrees forward while texting, you are putting 60 pounds of pressure on your neck! This results in neck pain that is so common, it is now a recognized condition called "text neck"! To avoid text neck, text with the phone out in front of you and at eye level. Or if you are reading in bed or on the couch, put a pillow in your lap so your arms and the reading material are elevated. Specialty catalogs offer book

*(continued on next page)*

*(continued from previous page)*

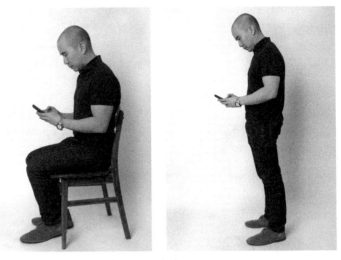

Improper device use

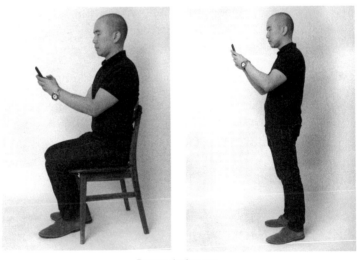

Proper device use

supports that permit you to prop a book on a table for hands-free reading. Utilize similar props for your devices—even the cover for your iPad helps tilt the screen upward!

**FAQ: Is it okay to adjust my own neck?** The answer is no! By twisting your neck improperly, you can really overstretch the ligaments. If you are someone who feels the need to adjust your neck, seek out a professional to do so.

## CHOKE POINT #5: Temporal Mandibular Joint or TMJ

The jaw joint happens to be one of the most important joints in the entire body. It is where the mandible (your jaw) meets the temporal bone (a bone in your skull right above your ear), hence the name the temporal mandibular joint. There are about a half dozen muscles that connect throughout the jaw. These muscles need to be in balance with equal pull from each of these muscles. When the TMJ joint does not move in a synchronous or smooth manner, a myriad of symptoms will appear, including jaw pain, headaches, ear pain, and yes, back pain—in both the lower and upper back and shoulders. Typically, patients with TMJ-related back pain will report feeling stiff and tight all throughout the back and spine. They will also frequently exhibit an inability to adequately open their mouth and may find that their jaw clicks or sometimes gets stuck in position. A TMJ sufferer may also clench or grind his or her teeth, either when awake or sleeping. Clenching your teeth while you are awake is a normal physiologic reaction to stress and is part of a body's natural "fight or flight" mechanism. The problem is that a stressed TMJ releases hormones such as cortisol, which raises the inflammatory factor in the body. This results in fatigue and pain, not just to the TMJ joint but to your entire body.

If you answered "yes" to these questions in the Back Pain Inflammatory Index, TMJ is probably a cause for your pain.

- ▸ Do you have a difficulty chewing hard foods?

- ▸ Are you only chewing foods on one side of your mouth?

- ▸ Are you aware that you clench your teeth?

- ▸ Has your dentist ever noted that you grind your teeth?

- ▸ Do you suffer from headaches more than once every two weeks?

- ▸ Does your jaw click when talking or chewing?

These self-tests are effective in confirming at TMJ diagnosis:

1. Open your mouth as wide as you can and see how many fingers stacked horizontally you can fit inside. You should be able to fit at least three fingers at one time.

**2.** Sit up tall and turn your head. Note how far you can turn. Bring your head back to center, then turn again with your mouth open. If you can see further with your mouth open, you know that your jaw is restricting your overall body's function.

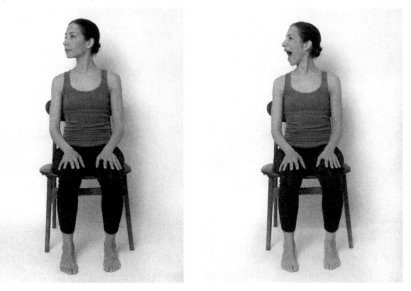

Now that you are aware of your TMJ issue, be cognizant of your clenching. Soft tissue or muscular techniques such as stretches and massage work well to balance these muscles and keep them loose. You can

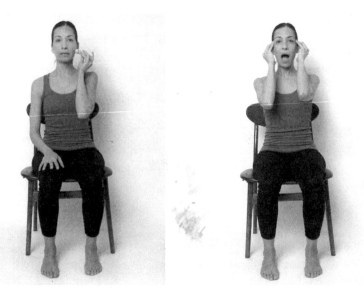

do one on your own by placing your hands gently on the TMJ muscles and opening and closing your jaw. Do the same stretch while putting your hands on your temporalis muscle. Do ten reps, three times a day. You can also give your jaw and the temporalis a good massage by using a micromassager for one or two minutes, as shown at the bottom of the facing page. The one I use is a Rolyan® Micro Mini Massager from Patterson Medical

> ▶ **MOUTH GUARD TIP:** Over-the-counter mouth guards can be bought at any local drugstore; but, if you want a customized mouth guard, try a Pro Teeth guard. Proteethguard.com is an online dental lab that works directly with the customer and has a great money back guarantee, allowing you to get a customized mouth guard significantly cheaper than at a dentist's office. If you need additional help, your dentist can give you individualized attention and make one for you.

Backbridge™ is also important to integrate into your daily routine for this kind of pain because a good amount of TMJ discomfort could be a result of poor posture in the neck and shoulders. Improving your posture goes a long way in reducing the tension in the jaw.

Remember, TMJ is often caused by stress, so stress management techniques tend to be helpful.

Combined, these TMJ solutions will help you target the source of your TMJ and find relief within three weeks!

Little known tidbit for braces and Invisalign® wearers: When trying to straighten your teeth, you are also altering your jaw alignment. Be aware of how your neck, shoulders, and jaw feel when you are shifting your bite. Braces and Invisalign® could be the mysterious cause of your back and or neck pain. With braces, you don't have a choice, but when using Invisalign®, you may need to slow down the progression of your trays to protect the mouth from intense shifting and allow the TMJ joint to adjust to the changes in the bite. With both, you should be integrating more TMJ stretches.

. . .

I WENT TO *Dr. Sinett complaining of headaches, neck and shoulder tightness, and some overall achiness. I was under a lot of stress and was waking up feeling sore throughout my entire body—almost as if I had a really hard workout, but I hadn't. My mouth and teeth also hurt. After touching my jaw, Dr Sinett surmised that I was clenching my teeth a lot. I was told to try a mouth guard, which I got from the drugstore and molded myself. After wearing it for one night I couldn't believe the difference. My symptoms were significantly better. I wear my mouth guard now every night, and it has made a huge improvement in my life. I urge anyone who may feel similarly to try it—it may be the best $20 you ever spend.*

*Isabella Ibragnov*

# Lighten Your Load

While the shoulders aren't a "choke point," there's an additional way that we are majorly throwing ourselves out of whack, and it's coming from the shoulder. You know your oversized handbag or that gym duffel you lug around all day? Carrying a too-heavy bag can cause your shoulders to become uneven. This is most common in women, whose large purses are a part of their everyday routine. When carrying a heavy tote on your arm or shoulder, you actually elevate the working shoulder, throwing your spine and overall sense of balance off kilter. It's even worse than if you are using a cell phone without a headset! You are also at risk for "bag jerk," the term I use when a bag slides off of your shoulder abruptly, causing your body to twist and strain and leading to painful neck and shoulder injuries.

This kind of damage can be comparable to a painful sports injury, and if not remedied, can create a long-term back problem. Here are some general guidelines to help keep your sack shoulder-friendly:

• The American Chiropractic Association recommends that a handbag weigh no more than ten percent of its owner's body weight. Choose a lightweight bag and clean it out frequently to avoid the build-up of junk you don't need.

• Try switching hands and shoulders when carrying your handbag. This will balance your "workout."

• If you carry two bags (a purse and a gym back or a briefcase and a bag), carry them on opposite sides to balance out the weight.

• To prevent bag jerk, make sure your bag has a wide, comfortable shoulder strap that has some grip to it (many shoulder straps now come with a rubberized coating to prevent slipping). Also, always adjust the shoulder strap—the height should be no lower than your hip so the bag does not impede your normal walk. If you have especially narrow shoulders, gravity may always win and bag jerk might be unavoidable. In this case, choose a messenger style bag that you can wear across your body, a traditional briefcase, or bag that does not go over the shoulder.

# 4

# THE ROLE OF POSTURE AND FLEXIBILITY

N ow that we have an introduction to the five "choke points" (and our bonus pain problem in the shoulders!), let's make sure we aren't missing two more things that are key to our bigger structural picture: posture and flexibility.

Good posture means that when a person is viewed from the side standing, he or she should have complete vertical alignment of the five choke points. You can ask your chiropractor to do a complete examination to help you in your self-diagnosis. Here's how I assess posture:

**Ear Levels:** Uneven ears suggest a head tilt, which can create discomfort in the upper neck.

**Symmetrical Jaw:** An asymmetrical jaw can be the cause of headaches and neck, jaw, and ear pain!

**Straight curve of the neck:** Carrying your head too far forward weighs poorly on those muscles!

**Shoulder balance and rotation:** Uneven or forward-pulling shoulders lead to neck and shoulder pain. There are many nerves that exit the neck, pass through the shoulder area, and supply the elbows and hands, so imbalanced shoulder heights can also cause carpal tunnel or wrist and forearm pain!

**Arm hang:** It's important to note if the arms are symmetrical when they are down at your sides and if the hands are rotated excessively inward or outward, which would suggest a shoulder imbalance.

**Pelvis and Hips:** Differing heights or rotation affect the low back.

**Knees:** Bowed or asymmetrical knees indicates lack of alignment while standing.

**Feet:** The nature of the arches show where an imbalance lies!

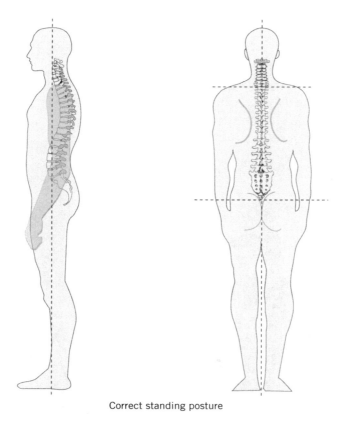

Correct standing posture

When doing a structural evaluation, the actual symptoms are secondary to getting the body in structural alignment. Remember, everything is related! After proper alignment is achieved, people are amazed at how many other symptoms go away.

# THE TREACHEROUS FORWARD HEAD TILT

The Forward Head Tilt. Cue the ominous music!

Many of the patients I see suffer from neck pain brought on by poor postural habits, like reading the paper or driving a car with their heads thrust forward (modern life has given us lazy necks!). Remember, this puts stress on the spine, resulting in dysfunction, and varying levels of pain or discomfort, from headache to back pain, to spinal stenosis or osteoarthritis (a progressive breakdown of cartilage that protects and cushions the joints). Eventually, this can lead to bone rubbing on bone, an exceedingly painful condition that can limit a person's overall quality of life.

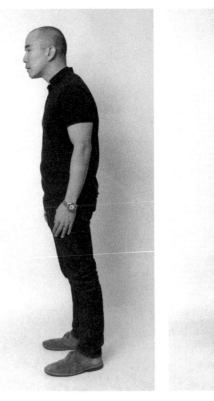

Foreward head tilt                    Correct posture

Imagine that your head is a bowling ball (the weight is actually quite similar!), and your neck is a stick trying to hold it up. If the ball pitched forward, it would fall off the stick. Luckily, this can't happen to your head. But, when your head slips forward, neck and shoulder tightness occur because the muscles have to strain to hold on to the head.

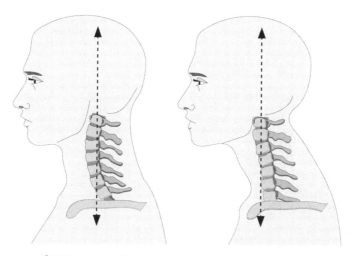

Correct neck position          Incorrect neck position

The greater the forward head carriage, the bigger the pain (and arthritis) in your neck. Stretches and exercises, including those with the Backbridge™, as well as ergonomic repositioning and chiropractic adjustment can all help in correcting this postural problem.

## Redefining Backbreaking Work

One of the main causes of chronic musculoskeletal pain is our sedentary lifestyle. Sitting exerts 30% more pressure on your spine than standing, so work that looks light and easy, such as sitting at a desk all day, is actually backbreaking. Add in a car or train commute that involves more sitting, and your body is paying the price!

I call this condition *disuse syndrome*. If you don't give your muscles something to do, they get weaker and smaller. If you sit around, your joints lose lubrication and age faster. And if you don't keep a healthy, aligned spine, you lose energy and balance, and over time, your joints degenerate.

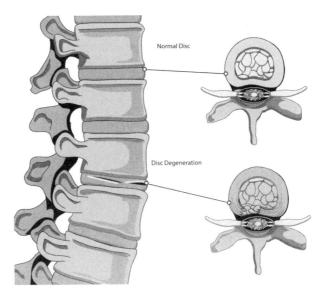

Normal Disc

Disc Degeneration

Degeneration of the spine

## QUICK QUIZ

Who do you think has more back pain? The farmer, who spends his day plowing a field and shoveling manure, or the office worker, who works from a desk eight hours a day?

The answer is the office worker.

The real backbreaking jobs are the ones that keep us seated, doing small movements over and over. While a farmer can certainly overdo lifting or pulling, thus creating a sprain or strain injury, farming allows a person to move his or her body in all different directions, keeping an overall balance in the farmer's body and building up strength evenly.

# Sitting Is Sucking the Life Out of You!

I've mentioned the hot catchphrase that doctors everywhere are spouting: "Sitting is the new smoking." It's true. A sedentary lifestyle affects your bones, muscles, and organs and can even shorten your life. Here's how:

## Organs

### HEART

Your blood flow slows during a long sit, so fatty acids can more easily clog the heart. That's why sedentary folks are two times more likely to develop cardiovascular disease.

### PANCREAS

Insulin isn't as productive in the cells of idle muscles, so the pancreas has to produce higher levels of it. Overproduction of insulin can cause diabetes and encourages cell growth, which can lead to several types of cancers, including colon and breast.

## Muscles

### HIPS

Sitters often suffer from tight hips because sitting doesn't allow you to extend the hip flexors.

### GLUTES

Strong glutes allow you to have a powerful stride. Sitting doesn't work your glutes in any way, which often decreases your overall stability.

## Circulation

Sitting reduces the speed of circulation, causing blood to pool in the legs. Varicose veins, blood clots and swollen feet and ankles can all arise as a result of this poor circulation.

Movement encourages blood flow to the brain, allowing brain and mood boosters to be released. Sitting for a long time can slow brain function!

## Bones

Physical activity stimulate lower body bones to grow dense and strong. Sitting lends itself to softer bones, making you more susceptible to osteoporosis.

And now for THE BACK . . .

## Neck

If most of your day is spent hunched at your desk, your neck is likely craned forward, too. Add in a few phone calls, holding the phone between your shoulder and ear while you type, and you are impacting your cervical vertebrae and creating a dangerous imbalance.

## Shoulders

Your bad posture overextends the shoulders, making them stiff and sore!

## Spine

Spines that sit too much become rigid and inflexible, putting you at risk for injury even during a simple activity, like bending down.

## Discs

Specifically, the discs in your spine get squashed when you sit, and the collagen around all of your supporting tendons and ligaments begins to harden. Sitters are at particularly heightened risk for herniated lumbar discs, caused by the pull of the upper body as it forward hunches.

## Lifestyle

People who watched seven or more hours of TV a day over the course of an eight-year study were at significantly higher risk of death (61%) than those who watched less than an hour a day.

Exercise is essential to staving off back pain. You don't have to start by running a marathon. UCLA conducted a study on the effects of back exercises and found that walking for a total of three hours per week helped relieve more back pain than doing low back exercises. The positive impact seemed to come not only from the physical benefits of exercise but also the relaxation aspect of walking.

# THE THREE-WEEK TEST

If you would say you live a sedentary lifestyle with frequent long days sitting, here is my three-week challenge: exercise three to four times a week for the next three weeks. Going for a brisk walk, taking a swim, or playing a round of tennis is all you need to get your muscles working in a bigger way and refresh and strengthen your muscles. Thirty minutes is all you need, and the time should be broken into three equal parts: warm-up, training, and cool-down. This simple workout method removes the shock factor to your muscular system and back. By warming up and cooling down properly, your muscles will be more flexible, which will ensure better posture and prevent over-contraction.

## Sleep with Proper Posture!

If you are waking up tight and stiff every morning, your mattress may be the culprit. One study conducted by Oklahoma State University researchers and reported in the *Journal of Chiropractic Medicine* revealed that subjects who suffered from persistent back pain found immediate and significant relief by switching to a new mattress and that the improvements persisted past the initial switch. The study also found that subjects who slept on mattresses that were at least five years old were significantly more likely to suffer from back pain and stiffness.

You can and should be promoting spinal health while you sleep! The combination of a medium-firm mattress and correct pillow can make a big difference in maintaining all of the curves of the spine—the neck, the mid-back, and the lower back. Medium-firm mattresses give support but also conform to the body, which is less stressful to the spine.

*Do you need a new mattress? Here's an easy-to-remember ABC to help you decide.*

**A (AGE):** Has your mattress had more than eight years of nightly use?

**B (BEAUTY):** Does your mattress have stains, soil, or tears? Does it sag?

**C (COMFORT):** When you lie down and concentrate on the comfort of your mattress, does it feel good or is it beginning to hollow out and sag in places?

> **TIP:** When buying a new mattress or testing your own for support, try this simple support test: Lie flat on your back on the mattress and place your hand under the small of your back. How much space is there? You should be able to move your hand around!

Before purchasing a new mattress, make sure the store has a flexible return policy and will allow you to take the mattress for a test drive. A thirty-day trial period allows you substantial time to listen to your body and see how the mattress is affecting it. Do you wake up feeling relaxed and refreshed? Do you feel as if you had a good night's sleep? If you don't, send it back! If you keep it, remember to rotate and reverse the mattress every six months to even out the wear.

A great way to try out mattresses is to sleep around! This advice may or may not be what you think! Ultimately, pay attention when you are in hotels or staying as a guest in other's homes, and listen to your body and your back when you wake up the next morning. If you wake up feeling refreshed, ask yourself, "Was that mattress firmer than mine? Does it have a cushy pillow top that made it softer than what I am used to?" Your body will tell you what kind of mattress you should commit to!

## How To Sleep

Patients often ask, "What is a proper sleeping position? Side, back, or stomach?"

If you are able to fall asleep, that generally means you are comfortable. Prescribing a sleep position would only make you uncomfortable and prevent natural habits. However, if you are suffering from back pain, here are ideal sleep positions:

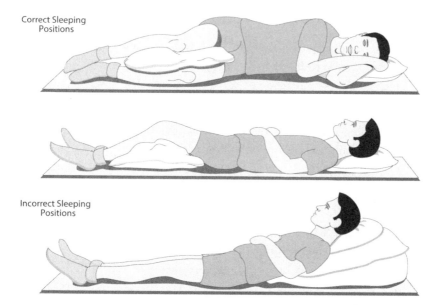

Correct Sleeping Positions

Incorrect Sleeping Positions

▶ **TIP:** Sleep with one pillow! Using multiple pillows lifts your neck to a stressful angle, preventing the area from relaxing. One pillow—and my personal choice, a water pillow—is the best option to prevent back and neck pain. Water pillows are dynamic, so no matter how you move, the supportive aspects of the pillow adjusts right with you!

## DON'T FLAKE ON FLEXIBILITY

Flexibility is vital to our health, but even people who exercise regularly prove to be low on flexibility. Flexibility helps you maintain good muscle tone, stay balanced, and age better. Oh yes—and maintain a healthy back! People with a strong back likely have good spinal flexibility.

Here are a few tests to gauge your flexibility:

- ► Can you touch your toes? If not, can you touch your ankles?

- ► Can you clap your hands behind your neck?

- ► Can you drop your chin to your chest?

- ► Can you put your head back and look up without it hurting?

▸ When you bend to the side, can you touch the sides of your knees?

▸ When standing with your feet pointing ahead of you, extend your arms and twist to the left. Then twist to the right. You ought to be getting to approximately the same point on both sides.

▸ Try bending your head to the left; then to the right. Ideally, you want to be able to get your ear almost to your shoulder on each side without raising your shoulder.

## Five tips for achieving optimal flexibility

1. **Adopt a safe and effective stretching program. Consistency is key.** Building or maintaining optimum flexibility requires regular stretching. You can't expect to be flexible if you only stretch once in a while. It also helps you de-stress, collect your thoughts, and tune into your body.

2. **"No pain, no gain" doesn't apply to stretching.** Pain when stretching means the muscle fibers are strained. These fibers can create scar tissue as the area heals, which increases the risk of problems and stiffness in the future. This is the opposite effect you want to achieve by stretching!

3. **Your stretching routine doesn't have to take a long time.** Between 10 and 15 minutes is sufficient time to thoroughly stretch your entire body. Do not rush through the stretches. Taking time with each position is more effective and reduces the risk of injury.

4. **Never end a workout without a stretch.** Many people believe the misconception that it is more important to stretch before exercising than it is to stretch after. Actually, stretching too much before working out can increase the risk of straining or tearing your muscles. It is much better to do a light cardio warm-up first and save the more aggressive stretching for afterward. If you do this consistently, you will also reduce any feelings of soreness.

5. **Practice balanced stretching.** Stretch each area of the body equally. Stretching one area more than another can actually create an imbalance in your flexibility!

The Backbridge™ is my innovative way to achieve optimal back flexibility. See pages 99-112 for more on flexibility and the Backbridge™.

• • •

*Dear Dr Sinett,*

*I want to thank you profusely for the Backbridge™. After years of seeing a chiropractor, exercise, medications, and visits to specialists after an MRI showed herniated discs, I could barely drive to the store to buy groceries. I could not sleep or concentrate. I was depressed and on meds. I was considering surgery.*

*The Backbridge™ is a miracle. I have been pain free for six weeks.*

*My energy has returned. I feel ten years younger, and I am again a happy smiling drugless man.*

*THANK YOU, THANK YOU, THANK YOU. You have made a huge difference in my life.*

*Best,*
*Mikail Collins*

## Structural Evaluation Checklist

In this chapter, you have learned about the global/compensatory issues rooted in the five "choke points" that cause back pain, as well as the contribution of poor posture and inflexibility. Let's review the ways to identify your global/compensatory issues:

**FEET:** An imbalance in the feet may be causing back pain if:

- ▶ Your feet hurt on a regular basis.
- ▶ Your shoes do not wear down evenly right to left.
- ▶ Footwear choices affect the way your body feels.

**PELVIS:** If your hands do not align when you place them on your hips, your pelvis is off balance. It may be difficult to tell, so check yourself out in the mirror—or even ask your tailor! Sitting on your wallet is one of the most common causes of pelvic misalignment in men!

**CORE/MID-THORACIC**: If you suffer from back pain and spend long hours at a computer desk or commuting in a car, you can safely assume you have pain coming from your core/mid-thoracic!

**NECK:** Tightness in the neck and shoulders or a pressing need to crack your neck is a sure sign that the neck is causing you problems.

**TMJ:** Your jaw may be causing you pain if:

- ▶ You clench your teeth from stress.
- ▶ You grind your teeth at night.
- ▶ You chew on one side.
- ▶ You have difficulty chewing hard food.

A lot of times, it's the little things compounded over time that create pain. Any of the above can cause poor posture and throw your alignment off, causing a structural issue. Lack of flexibility or improper stretching, for example, can cause a simple issue to turn into something much bigger. Getting to the root of the structural cause is essential in finding the right solution, so be diligent in your self-assessment of these points! What's also essential is being consistent in your treatment. My tips are easy to do—but they are also easy NOT to do. You have to remember that these tips are your treatment, and schedule them into your day until they become habit. Remember, three weeks forms a habit.

# 5

# CORE IMBALANCE

At first glance, the administrative assistant and the fitness trainer who both visited my office appeared to have nothing in common. Tracy, a middle-aged office worker, spent a minimum of 40 hours a week at her desk, bent over a computer or crunched up taking phone messages. Her commute to and from the office put her on a city bus for about 25 minutes each morning and evening. She did make time to exercise regularly, but was still suffering from lower back pain.

Kyle's lifestyle was in sharp contrast to Tracy's. He was a personal trainer in his early thirties who spent all day at a gym teaching spin and other fitness classes and working with individual clients. He came to me for help with back and shoulder pain, as well as debilitating migraine headaches.

The commonality between these patients? Despite having very different symptoms, they both had core imbalance. Ultimately, both Kyle and Tracy spent too much time working their abs. While Tracy's job doesn't sound as if it entails much abdominal work, the very act of being hunched over (at a computer or in a bus) all day mean that her abdomen was almost always in a state of crunch with her muscles contracted for much of the day. Kyle was doing lots of crunches and sit-ups and curling over his bike in spin class. Whether a person's abs are pulled tight because of bad posture, long periods of sitting, or physical exercise, the results are the same: core imbalance.

# WHAT IS CORE IMBALANCE?

Core imbalance is the condition of excessive compression, which results in the spine curving forward in a C-like shape. It can be caused by many everyday activities, such as sitting at a computer, reading in bed, or driving a car, which is why many people with nine-to-five jobs feel back and neck pain. It can also be self-imposed in our quest for six-pack abs by doing crunches or other improper core training (though many trainers don't know these exercises qualify as improper fitness!). Core imbalance is extremely prevalent across all ages and all demographics, especially now that we are a society that is hunched over our devices for much of the day!

Tension headaches, temporal mandibular joint (TMJ) problems, stiff necks, elbow, wrist, and arm pain, knee pain, lower back pain, dizziness, difficulty breathing, and poor digestion are just a few of the complaints arising from core imbalance. It can even lead to arthritis and degeneration of the spine.

For most people, the problem is your core. In treating my patients with core imbalance, I've learned two rules of thumb about combating back pain that stems from misuse of the abdominals:

- ► For every forward movement, there needs to be a counter movement. It's vital that we put extension into our routine to counteract the flexion, or crunching and hunching, we do all day. When your chest is open and uplifted, as it is when you are sitting up straight, your heart, lungs, and other bodily systems have less pressure on them, and you experience an increase in oxygen intake, improved blood and lymph supply, better digestion, better flexibility, and an overall improvement in health. With regular use of my anti-core-imbalance exercises, you should feel an expansion of the chest and relief in the back.

- ► Every time you contract a muscle, you need to be sure to relax it. As a result of stress or bad habits, many people contract certain muscles but never allow them the opportunity to relax. Bodybuilders are frequently incapable of turning their heads fully because their muscles are so tight; it's as if they were in a straitjacket. A similar sensation may happen after a day of intense business meetings. You need to find a way to let those muscles release.

The Deep Breath Test gives you a better understanding of compression and expansion and can help you relax when you need to. Here's how to do it:

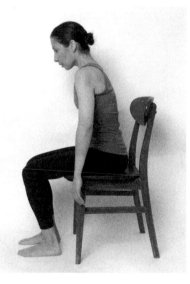 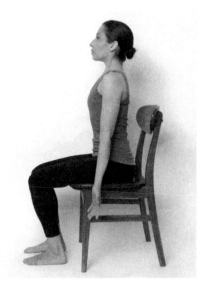

**1.** Slouch in your chair. Let your arms hang down. They will naturally rotate inward. Try to take a deep breath.

**2.** Now sit up tall. Extend both of your arms out at your sides (like airplane wings) and take a deep breath).

**3.** Try it one more time, this time with your arms straight up.

As you can see, you can take a much deeper breath simply by improving your posture, which in turn opens your chest. If you retrain your muscles, you can breathe more deeply and easily and help yourself find more relaxation within your stressful day.

## Do You Have Core Imbalance? Take the Core Imbalance Test!

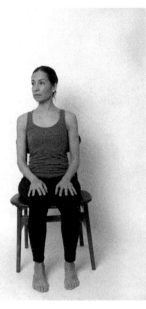 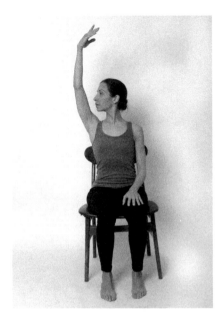

**1.** Sit in an ordinary chair, facing forward, with your feet on the floor. Now turn your head to the right and note how far you can see behind you.

**2.** Turn back to your starting position and lift your right arm above your head. Now turn your head to the right again.

If you can see farther with your arm raised, then you have a core that is out of balance.

Why does this test work? By elevating your arm, you are stretching your abdominal muscles, allowing a release to happen. If you need the release to gain vision, this means that your abs are the culprit for your decreased range of motion!

## THREE WEEK TREATMENT FOR CORE IMBALANCE

My two-tiered approach to correcting core-imbalance will help you find a little relief right away and you will feel almost completely pain-free if you do the stretch and exercises every day for three weeks.

## TIER 1: The Backbridge™

After seeing many patients with core imbalance, I started to study the benefits of extension therapy, but it wasn't until I began working with a patient who happened to be an ESPN fitness model that I had my "aha" moment. She was the picture of health but, like Kyle, was suffering terribly with neck and back pain. While I was taking down her case history, she said that she did thousands of sit-ups and crunches on her fitness show. *What could I do to put immediate extension into her back?* I wondered. I grabbed one of the big exercise balls we had in our therapy room and had her lay on her back and stretch over it. To her surprise and mine, after stretching over the ball for a few minutes, she felt significantly better. I then took the ball and went to show my father, whom I was still working alongside at the time, what I had discovered. He proceeded to lie over the ball—only to fall off of it!

Off to the drawing board I went. I wanted to design a product that was more stable and would put similar extension into one's spine, but in a gradual and safe manner. After years of tinkering, I finally perfected it and created a product called Backbridge™. With its different levels, Backbridge™ allows anyone to use it comfortably by progressively undoing all of the forward hunch that our body gets. Two minutes, twice a day on the Backbridge™ is enough to let the spine curve backward slightly, extending and loosening the back muscles, opening the chest, and permitting deeper breathing.

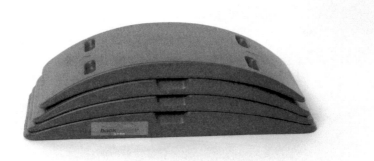

This stretch can be done on an exercise ball (also called a physio ball or a yoga ball) as first tested with my patient. However, the ball lacks stability, and while this is one of its benefits when working other parts of the body, when lying on your back with the purpose of back release, it is much more helpful and effective not to be wobbling side to side! If you don't have a yoga ball or a Backbridge™, you can also simply roll up a beach towel to create a cylinder about 12 inches long and four to five inches in diameter, depending on your current level of flexibility. Place the towel on the floor, then lie down with the towel in line with your spine and allow your head to rest on the floor with no strain on the neck.

The Backbridge™ ultimately is most effective since it allows you to gradually increase your back flexibility by adding levels of arch, while the ball and towel alternatives only give you one stretch. I often recommend that patients try at-home extension methods to start. When they begin to see the relief, they usually want a Backbridge™!

No matter which tool you are using, when lying on your support, extend both of your hands above your head, allowing the maximum amount of stretch and chest opening. If this is uncomfortable, place your hands behind your head, across your chest, or alongside you.

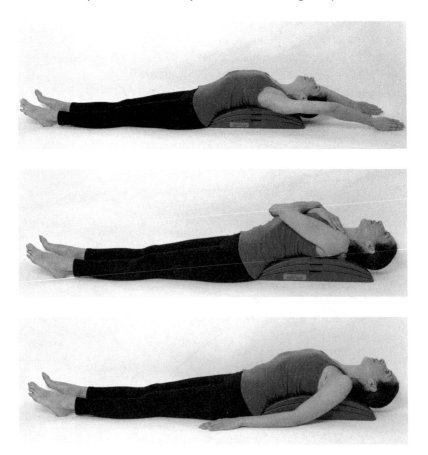

Start with just 30 seconds a day and gradually increase to two to three minutes a day. Many people who have core imbalance are extremely tight and starting with short time periods allows you to introduce the counter-stretch without pulling the muscle or causing other injury.

When your time is up, roll to your side and slowly come up to a sitting position. You will find a little bit of relief the first time you do this stretch, but do it every day for three weeks, and you will feel better throughout an entire day. This Tier One stretch may be all that you need. Just two minutes in the morning and two minutes at night has changed thousands of people's lives. It is that easy, and all it requires from you is consistency.

So why is there a Tier Two solution at all? I created Tier Two, which follows, after seeing that my patients wanted to do more with the Back-bridge™. Bringing the Backbridge™ into your workouts allows you to exercise without putting your body into a forward hunch, and my exercise routine ensures that you are strengthening all of your core muscles so that you have strong, balanced abs!

## TIER 2: Exercises for Strong, Balanced Abdominals

Over-exercising, under-exercising, or doing the wrong exercises that put more forward flexion into our abs can cause imbalance, which eventually results in back pain. Integrating the right exercise in moderation will not only help you fight core imbalance but will also allow you to get a firm,

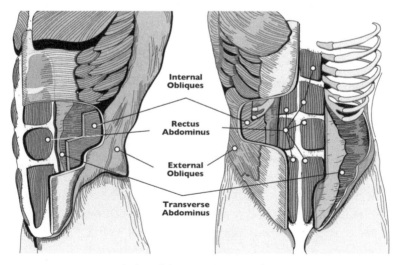

A view of the abdominal muscles

fit stomach, too. These exercises are easy to do and take less than ten minutes a day! In conjunction with the Backbridge™ or other extension stretch, you will strengthen your core muscles the right way, allowing you to hold yourself up with better posture and eliminating some of that forward hunch.

This program targets all three abdominal groups:

**The Transverse Abdominus:** The flat, triangular muscle that pulls the abdominal wall inward and acts as an internal girdle to stabilize the spine. It is the key to your core stability.

**The Rectus Abdominus:** This muscle is responsible for allowing us to bend our trunks forward; it also brings the ribs closer to the pubic bone. This is the muscle that gets overworked from crunching postures and activities. It has no stabilizing effect on the back.

**The Internal and External Obliques:** These muscles permit us to twist our trunks: the external oblique muscle is the outermost muscle that covers the side of the abdomen, and the internal oblique is smaller and thinner and lies just within the external one, providing extra support for side-to-side movements.

## SIX MYTHS ON GETTING A SIX PACK

### MYTH 1
#### Strong Abs Means a Strong Back

"I need to work on my six pack" is something I hear all the time, especially as summer approaches. But actually, your abs are likely already too strong—even if you don't exercise regularly—from all of the hunching and forward flexion that is already in your daily lifestyle. This means that your strong core is out of balance with the rest of your muscles. It is hard to wrap our heads around this idea, especially when we are surrounded by trainers everywhere who still recommend sit-ups and crunches as the keys to obtaining a flat stomach. This just reinforces the misleading tenet that working out one part of your body will allow you to achieve great overall results.

It's up to you to remember the fine print: that results come only when used as part of a complete diet and exercise routine. The key to a strong back is *balanced* abdominal muscles, which comes from working your core equally with the other muscles in your body.

### MYTH 2
### A big gut is a sign of weak abs.

A T-shirt I once saw in an airport featured the saying, "This isn't a beer belly—just a protective covering for my rock-hard abs!" While big bellies indicate a high percentage of body fat, they don't indicate anything about abdominal muscle strength or weakness. Sumo wrestlers and large football players—and even some beer drinkers—don't have weak cores. Their muscles are just covered up with excess fat.

### MYTH 3
### Six-pack abs reflect good abdominal training.

Six-pack abs reflect nice-looking muscles, not necessarily properly functioning muscles. It is common for people with good-looking abs to suffer from back pain stemming from structural imbalance.

### MYTH 4
### Supporting your neck while doing sit-ups and crunches is the best way to protect your neck from injury.

Sit-ups and crunches are the worst exercises and should *never* be done. A common injury sustained during these exercises is "throwing" your neck out. Some people thought that this was caused by forgetting to support your neck, but actually, crunches and sit-ups cause the ab muscles to be pulled too tight, putting tremendous pressure on your neck. *This* is what causes neck pain.

### MYTH 5
### Pilates is a safe, low-impact way to exercise your stomach because it stretches and lengthens the spine, thus preventing injuries.

I have a good number of Pilates teachers as patients and I have seen how Pilates can cause pain. The Pilates Hundred places an

*(continued on next page)*

*(continued from previous page)*

overemphasis on developing abdominals by putting a person in the C position.

### MYTH 6

**An exercise mat and large ball are the two best pieces of equipment for getting a lean stomach.**

An overall good diet and exercise regimen are the keys to a lean stomach. Your sneakers are actually the best piece of equipment to use in order to lose that gut because they represent fat-burning aerobic exercise!

## EXERCISE ROUTINE FOR A BALANCED CORE

How do you get those flat abs without damaging your back and body? Here's how to build a six-pack, the right way! Most of these exercises require nothing at all, but an oversize exercise ball or the Backbridge™ is needed for some. You can purchase one for your home or do these exercises at a fitness center.

Start this program by doing one set of 12 repetitions on each side, but as you become stronger, you can increase to three sets of 12. The exercises are presented in level of difficulty, so if you are just starting out, start with the Beginner Level. Increase until you can do the maximum number of repetitions and then advance to the next level of difficulty. These exercises should be performed in conjunction with an active cardio program. I recommend doing what you enjoy, whether it be a swim, a walk, tennis, or a jog, and don't forget to include a warm up and a cool down.

. . .

DR. TODD PERIODICALLY *conducts Backbridge™ exercise sessions in his office that gently strengthen your core, back, and tone your body. I have had the pleasure of attending one of these sessions. It was one of the best work-outs that I have experienced. The exercises were gentle and simple enough for a 90-year-old woman to perform—and yet, I didn't know how hard I had worked until ten minutes after the class. I was energized and the burn was good!*

*Angela Spencer*

# START AND END YOUR ROUTINE WITH THE STANDING ABDOMINAL STRETCH

1. Stand with feet about hip distance apart, knees slightly bent.

2. Lift arms in front of you until they are extended straight overhead.

3. Bend back slightly, stretching the abs.

4. Repeat 12 times.

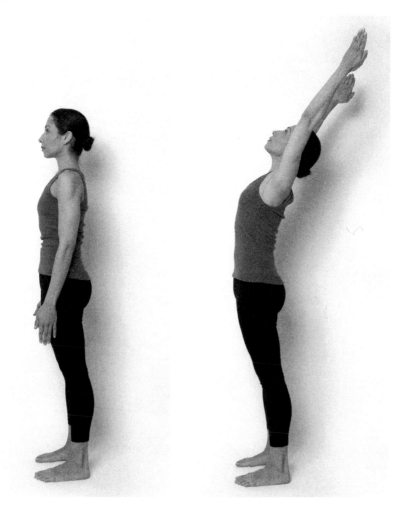

# ANTI-CORE IMBALANCE EXERCISES: Beginning Level

### The Skinnies

This exercise works the transverse abdomens.

1. Stand, sit, or lie down on your back and exhale completely.

2. Pull your navel in and up.

3. Hold for ten seconds and release.

4. Repeat 12 times.

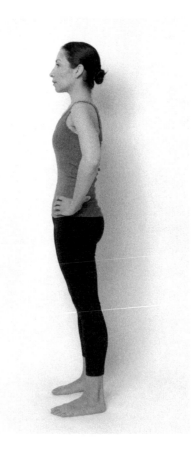

## Standing Side Twist

This exercise works the oblique muscles.

1. Stand with hands on hips.

2. With feet stationary, twist the abdomen to one side and hold for five seconds.

3. Twist the body to the other side.

4. Repeat 12 times.

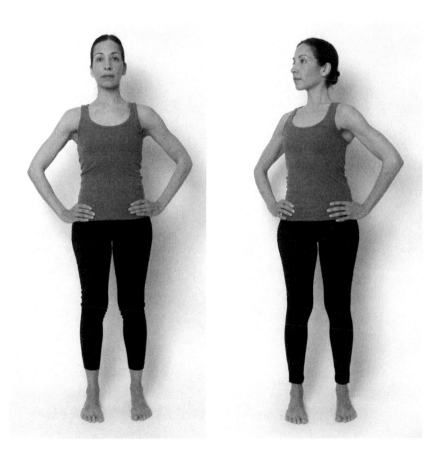

## Ball Roll Out

This exercise works the rectus abdominis.

1. Kneel in front of an oversize exercise ball.

2. Put your forearms on top of the ball and slowly roll it away from you, stretching and expanding your abdominal muscles as the ball rolls out.

3. Roll the ball back in with your arms in the same position.

4. Repeat 12 times.

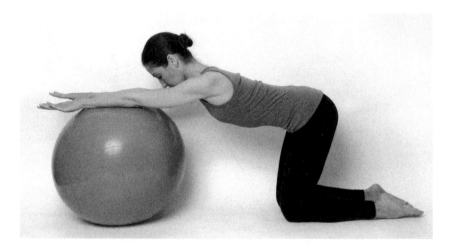

## Tummy Tucks

This exercise works both the transverse and the rectus-abdominis.

1. Lie on your back with your arms at your sides and your palms facing down.

2. Draw the navel in and down toward the floor.

3. Tilt your pelvis so your buttocks lift slightly off the floor.

4. Hold for ten seconds and release.

5. Repeat 12 times.

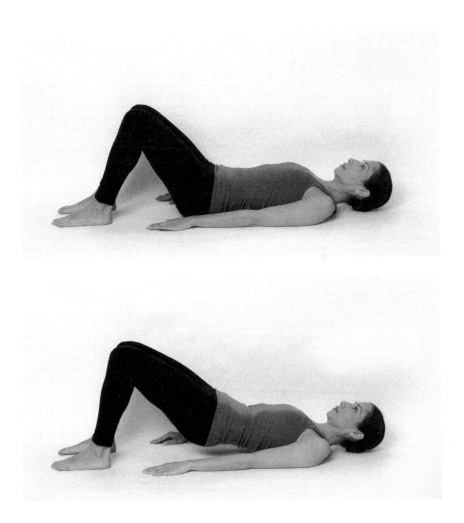

## ANTI-CORE-IMBALANCE EXERCISES:
## Intermediate Level

### Alternate Knee Tucks

This exercise works the rectus abdominis.

1. Lie on your back with your arms at your sides, your palms facing down, and your legs lying flat.

2. Bend the right knee, bringing it toward your chest.

3. Straighten the right knee, lowering it as you bring the left knee to your chest. (The motion resembles pedaling a bicycle.)

4. Repeat 12 times.

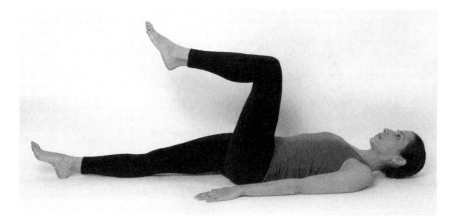

## Side Leg Raises

This exercise works the oblique muscles.

1. Lie on the floor on your side. Bend the arm beneath you and use it to support yourself with your torso lifted to a 45-degree angle.

2. Engage the side abdominals and lift the upper leg as far as you can but no further than 90 degrees.

3. Repeat 12 times.

4. Roll to your other side and repeat.

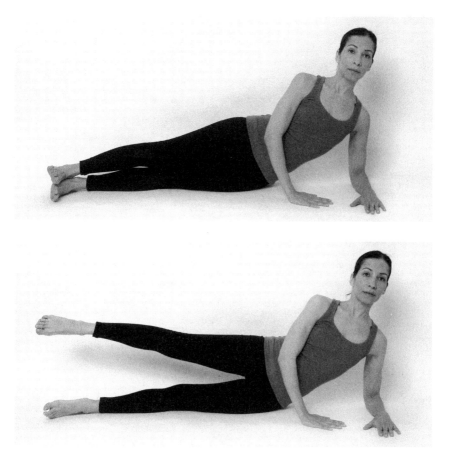

## Five-Second Plank

This exercise works both the rectus and transverse abdomens, building strength without the sense of failure many people experience when trying to do push-ups.

1. Assume basic push up position. Your hands should be flat on the floor directly under your shoulders, and your body should be raised in a straight line.

2. Pull the navel in toward the spine.

3. Hold for five seconds.

4. Fully release and relax onto the floor.

5. Repeat 12 times.

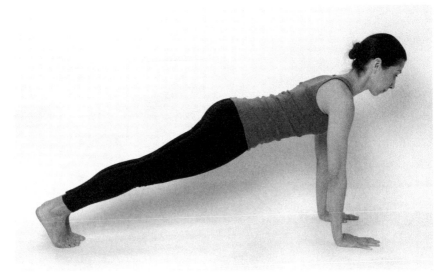

## Standing Twist with Ball (or Book)

This exercise works the oblique muscles. It requires something to hold, such as an oversize exercise ball, volleyball, hardcover book or a 12-ounce water bottle.

1. Stand with feet parallel, slightly apart.

2. Extend your arms straight in front of you, both hands holding the object out in front of your chest.

3. Twist your upper abdomen to one side.

4. Hold ten seconds.

5. Twist to the other side.

6. Repeat 12 times.

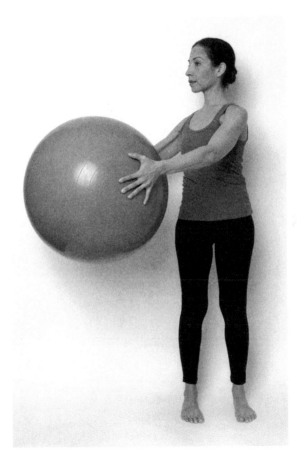

## ANTI-CORE-IMBALANCE EXERCISES: Advanced Level

### Single Leg Raise

This exercise works the rectus abdominis.

1. Lie on your back with your arms at your sides, your palms facing down, and your legs lying flat.

2. Engage the abdominals and lift one leg off the ground at approximately a 45-degree angle.

3. Slowly lower the leg.

4. Repeat on the other side.

5. Repeat 12 times.

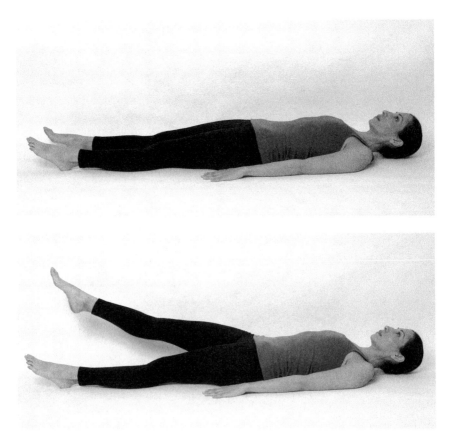

## Double Leg Raise

This exercise works the rectus abdominis.

1. Lie on your back with your arms at your sides, your palms facing down and your legs lying flat out.

2. Engage the abdominals and lift both legs slowly off the ground until they are at approximately a 45-degree angle. If this is challenging for you, put your hands under your lower back for support.

3. Slowly lower both legs to the floor.

4. Repeat 12 times.

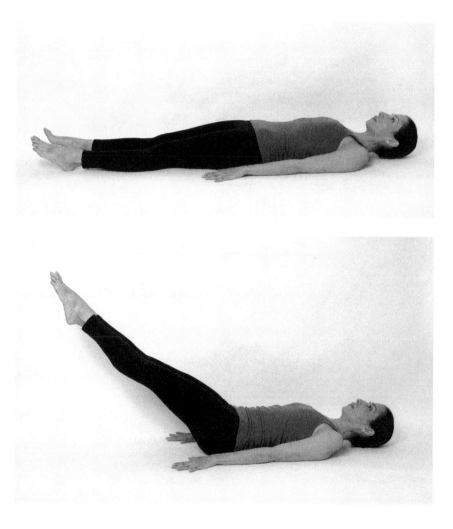

## Ball Lift

This exercise works the rectus abdominis. Requires a ball or small pillow (something that won't hurt if you drop it)

1. Lie on your back with your arms at your sides, your palms facing down, and your legs lying flat.

2. Place the object between your feet.

3. Lift the legs slowly (no higher than 90 degrees) while your feet continue to hold the object.

4. Slowly lower both legs to the floor.

5. Repeat 12 times.

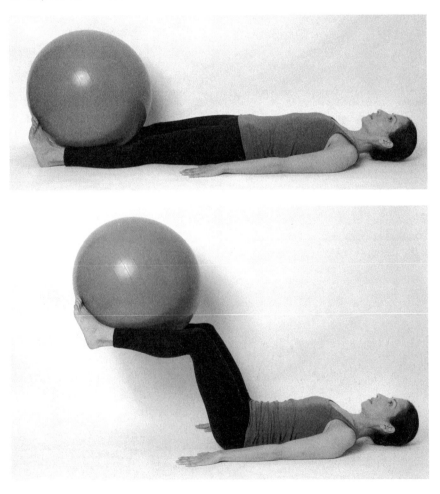

## Ten-Second Plank with Leg Lift

This exercise works the rectus abdominis.

1. Assume the basic push up position with hands flat on the floor directly under the shoulders and your body raised and in a straight line.

2. Pull the navel toward the spine.

3. Lift one leg straight up behind you.

4. Hold for ten seconds.

5. Repeat with the other leg.

6. Repeat 12 times.

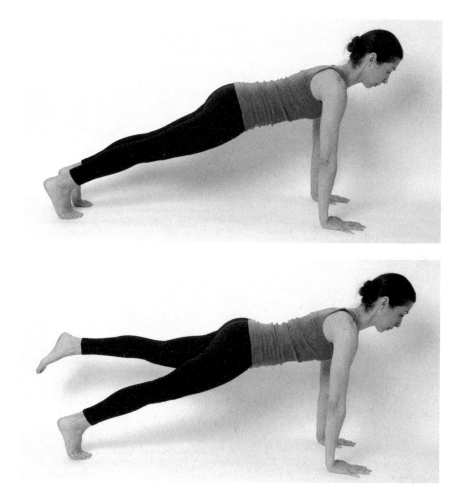

## Elbow Side Plank

This exercise works the oblique muscles.

**1.** Lie on your side, supporting your upper body on your forearm.

**2.** Engage the side abdominals and lift hips toward the ceiling, balancing on the side of one foot and the forearm of that same side.

**3.** Hold for ten seconds.

**4.** Repeat 12 times.

**5.** Roll to your other side and repeat.

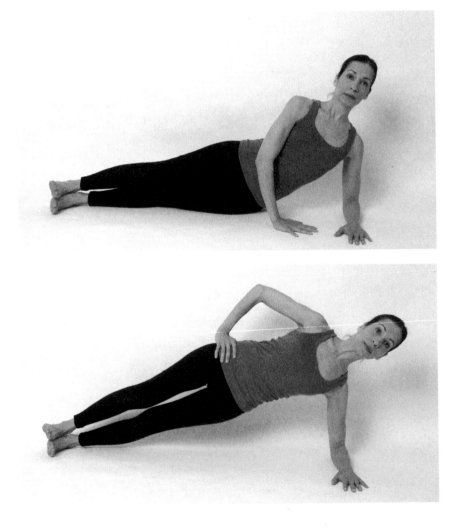

You can also perform this exercise using the Backbridge™ to rest your hip between sets or to elevate your feet or forearms for variation.

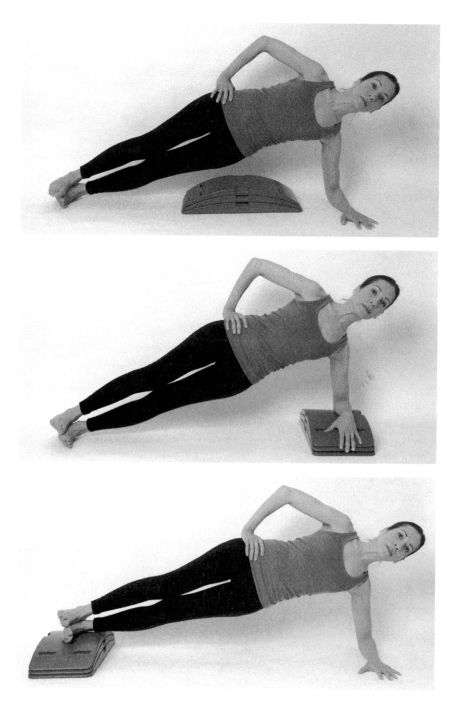

# WHAT IF WE TOOK CARE OF OUR BACKS LIKE WE DID OUR TEETH?

The dentists got it right: an ounce of prevention is worth a pound of cure. Dentists don't sit back and wait until a patient needs a root canal before they take action. Instead, they continually monitor, preventatively treat, and educate their patients on ways to take care of their teeth. What would happen if we took the same approach to caring for our spines and backs? It's surprising more people don't pose this question, considering how important our backs and spines are to our overall health! The truth is, if more people treated their back like they did their teeth, they'd feel a lot better and be a whole lot healthier.

## Setting the stage for preventative care

Americans have some of the best oral health in the world—and this did not happen overnight or by chance. The American Dental Association (ADA) is unified in its beliefs and standards of care for a patient's teeth at any age. Because of this unity, a strong message is conveyed: See your dentist for regular check-ups so you don't have to see him for something serious! Regular checkups that include x rays to make sure cavities aren't developing, dental cleanings to make sure that there is not too much tartar buildup, and assessments to make sure that a patient's mouth and teeth are looking generally straight and healthy are done. Numerous products and regimens were woven into our society's beliefs until they became the norm. In fact, dental care is so well engrained in our day-to-day life that most of us floss and brush at least twice a day. At-home dental care combined with regular in-office checkups and preventative treatments is an example of an ideal system of prevention.

## A strong foundation

People of all ages go to the dentist, floss, and brush. The importance of teeth does not diminish as we age—we should always take care of them. Just like our teeth affect our jaws, skulls, sinuses, nutrition, and even our hearts, our backs and spines are related to so much more than our posture or backaches. The back and spine not only help to keep the body in an upright position, they protect the nervous system. The nervous system includes the brain and spinal cord, controlling every single action in the entire body, from breathing to walking. Exiting from the spinal cord and spine are an intricate web of nerves that feed into all of the muscles and organs. Interference with any these nerves can lead to a myriad of symptoms, not limited to the classic "back pain."

By utilizing the dental approach with regard to the spine and back, people would get regular spine and back check-ups by a chiropractor, physical therapist, or orthopedist. These professionals would evaluate the functional level of the spine with a thorough check-up and then provide preventative treatments. In addition, instructions for at-home stretches and exercises would be provided, ensuring that in just minutes a day a patient could prevent or minimize back and spine troubles.

## Take a lesson from orthodontists

An orthodontist is a highly regarded dental specialist trained to treat misaligned teeth by looking at the teeth and jaw in a very dynamic manner and often utilizing dental braces to bring alignment back to the teeth. It is quite important to have straight, properly functioning teeth for many health reasons, in addition to cosmetic purposes. Even when orthodontic treatment is not covered by insurance, patients pay out of pocket because the importance of straight teeth has been ingrained in each of us from a young age.

We tend to deal with a crooked spine (scoliosis) much differently than the common sense dental model. Treatment for scoliosis is typically no treatment at all. Usually x rays are taken to measure the degree of crookedness. If the crookedness is not so severe, surgery is not needed, and no treatment is offered. This is not to say that treatments for scoliosis are not available or effective. Exercise, guided stretching, chiropractic treatments, and physical therapy can all help to prevent or reverse scoliosis! However, no consensus currently exists for treating scoliosis, let alone guidelines for which profession should be responsible for treating it. Chiropractors are the underutilized specialty along the lines of spinal orthodontics!

## The first step: Get away from the cliff

Though back and spine care is not near the preventative level of dental care, a good first step is avoiding the proverbial back pain cliff through regular check-ups with a chiropractor. Teetering on the edge of this cliff means one simple stress on your body can push you into the abyss of back pain. Regular check-ups create a larger space between your body and the edge of that dangerous cliff. It is the little things, like daily stretching and exercise, that make your body most resilient and prevent small issues from turning into big catastrophes.

## The second step: No excuses

If your teeth break or wear down, they can be mended or replaced. Unfortunately, dentures for the spine are not an option; artificial discs and vertebrae don't work very well and create many complications. You only get one spine, so take good care of it. And no, getting older is not a legitimate reason to lose back function or become less active. No matter what your age, activity level, flexibility, etc., there are gentle stretches and movements you can do to strengthen your back and prevent injury and pain.

## The final word

If you've ever had back pain, as most people have, you'll surely understand the appeal of prevention rather than treatment. Our spines should be regularly monitored and preventatively treated just like our teeth. At-home routines, the spinal equivalent to brushing and flossing, must become everyday habits for everyone. The Backbridge™ Solution, detailed in the following section, is your preventative (and curative) treatment, that can be done daily, in the same time it takes you to brush your teeth!

# 6

# THE BACKBRIDGE™ SOLUTION

## Regaining Back Flexibility and Vitality in Just Three Weeks

We know now that even activities that don't seem harmful, like sitting, or ones we think are actually healthful, like doing sit-ups, can put stress on our bodies and allow them to become stiff. In the structural prescription, I explained the positive impact my Backbridge™ (or other extension alternative) can have in relieving pain caused by too much flexion, or forward hunching, in your day. Lying over the Backbridge™ helps reduce soreness, tightness, or other feelings of pain caused not only by forward flexion, but also by aging, exercise, and daily life stressors. Stretching is a gentle exercise that should be done daily to help you loosen up stiff and tender muscles, relieve discomfort, regain the flexibility you had as a child, and even lengthen your life. The Backbridge™ enables you to stretch your back in ways that the exercise ball or a rolled up towel don't—and that's why I consider it a key part in your lifelong solution.

Why is it important to reclaim your flexibility? Our flexibility affects our ability to bend and move and impacts our overall vitality. In order to be truly healthy and fit, you need to have a balance of three fitness factors: 1) endurance, 2) strength, and 3) flexibility. As a doctor, I have seen too many patients and athletes who have more than adequate strength and aerobic function but who are severely lacking in flexibility.

# THE BENEFITS OF IMPROVED FLEXIBILITY

### Better posture

Having great flexibility means you'll also be able to stand up straighter, walk farther, and do more things with less pain. As we age, our joints and muscles stiffen, making it more difficult to perform various tasks, such as bending over, walking up steps, and even sitting. Better posture means less forward hunch, which means less back pain!

### Improved coordination prevents injury

Improved flexibility allows us to have better balance and coordination. Better balance and coordination means fewer falls—and fewer traumatic structural injuries!

### Improved Blood Circulation

Blood is pumped back to your heart through your veins by the squeezing and relaxing of skeletal muscles. Stretching helps relax your muscles, allowing circulation to improve. This has obvious benefits such as increased oxygen delivery, reduction in cramping, and an increased capacity for performance. In other words, better flexibility leads to better endurance and better recovery.

### The Backbridge™: The Sinett Uber Solution

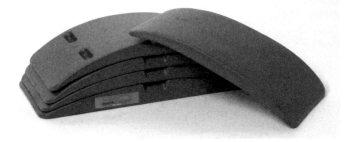

Backbridge™ is the perfect tool to help you improve the flexibility in your back for two main reasons:

1. Its arched, contoured design allows you to isolate the back muscles and results in a deeper stretch.

2. Its interlocking, stackable levels allow you to alter the intensity of any stretch. When you stretch at your own level of flexibility, you prevent injuries and discomfort from over-stretching. Without Backbridge™, stretches are static and essentially always the same. You wouldn't want to continually lift the same amount of weight or always do the same amount of aerobic exercise because your strength and endurance will plateau. Why would you always want to stretch the same? Being able to deepen your stretch allows your body to become stronger and more flexible, and Backbridge™ allows you to progress gradually and safely. This means the Backbridge™ can be used now, while you are in pain, and can still challenge you later, when you are pain-free!

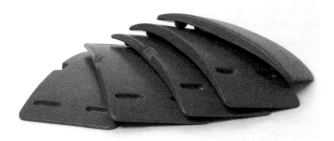

Here are tips to maximize the benefits of stretching your back with the Backbridge™:

**Move slowly!** It's not a race, so ease into each stretch to reduce the risk of over-stretching and subsequent injury.

**Stretch often.** Stretching increases the elasticity of your muscles, but you can't do it all in one 15 minute stretching workout. Stretching should be done frequently. Remember, one stretch won't make you flexible, just like going on one run won't make you aerobically fit! Make stretching your back a consistent part of your routine. You will feel relief if you commit to three weeks of stretching and sticking to it will prevent future pain.

**Breathe!** The key is to relax so you can achieve a better stretch. Remembering to breathe allows you to let go of the stress.

**It shouldn't be painful!** You shouldn't be grimacing in pain while stretching. Make sure to listen to your body and stay within your limits. While you should approach your boundaries, only do what you're actually capable of doing. Remember, if it hurts, don't do it. Pain is how your body tells you to stop moving a certain way. A stretch should be enjoyable—and should not induce any more back pain!

•   •   •

A DIFFERENT HOTEL *room every day, broken sleep on a moving tour bus, and countless hours spent in the air: this is what I called "home" as a professional in the touring music industry—and it had all taken its toll on me. Not only physically, but also mentally and emotionally.*

*While passing through New York on tour, a friend convinced me to meet with Dr. Sinett (more like dragged me kicking and screaming out of my hotel room). That day was the beginning of a new me.*

*Dr. Sinett was gentle and patient; and the friendship was instantaneous, as if we'd known one another for decades. He worked with me to address every aspect of my health, and my chronic neck and back pain saw marked improvement immediately. Dr. Todd sent me away with the Backbridge™, which has become my #1 travel companion. I have one for my traveling office, one for the tour bus, and one at home so that I never go without! And now, as a brand-new mother, the Backbridge™ has become even more invaluable to me.*

*Its omnipresence in my life tends to spark conversation and allow me the opportunity to pay it forward in the same way someone once did for me—from the artists that I work with, to friends, family, colleagues, and acquaintances, I love seeing others find the relief that I have found! The Backbridge™ has become a staple for artist friends on the road—and is the key to feeling great during a performance.*

*Meagan Strader*

## THE TOP TEN STRETCHES FOR A BETTER BACK

These ten back stretches will realign your spine and help correct postural imbalances that can be the underlying source of common back pain. The better your spinal alignment, the better your posture and flexibility, and the better your back will be—not to mention your overall quality of your life! Remember, these stretches are not only intended to help you recover from back pain, but to be free from it for life! If your commitment goes beyond the three weeks, so will your relief!

## 1. BACKBRIDGE™ EXTENSION

Previously referenced on page 76, this stretch is of utmost importance, in that it relieves the flexion of sitting and other activities that cause us to hunch! It is key to resolving your structural back pain. The stretch can

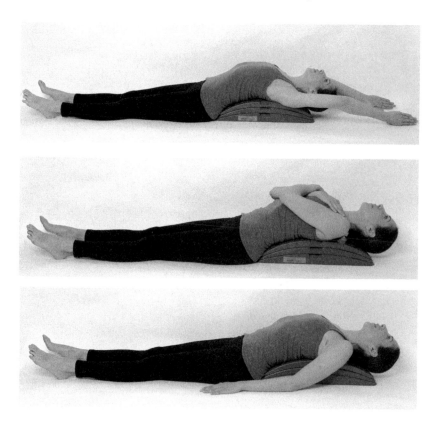

be done by placing the Backbridge™ on the floor, or if you are particularly tight and need to ease down to the ground, you may start by putting the Backbridge™ in bed or affixing it to your chair with the included strap.

First, sit at the base of the Backbridge™. Lie back so that the highest point of the Backbridge™ is between your shoulder blades and your head touches the floor. Rest your arms behind your head and hold this stretch for two minutes. Do this twice a day—once in the morning and once in the evening. Level 1 is the easiest and 5 is the hardest. Pick a level that is most comfortable for you. It should feel like a good stretch. After a few weeks, slowly progress to the next level.

Discovering this stretch sparked my understanding of forward flexion and its effect on the body. If you only do one thing in this entire book, the Backbridge™ Extension stretch is it! This alone can alleviate so much structural stress caused by sitting and hunching!

Remember, there are various ways you can position your arms while doing this stretch. If resting your arms behind your head doesn't feel good, try these variations and do what feels best for you!

## 2. SPINAL STRETCH

Lie on your back, placing the Backbridge™ under your knees. Reach your arms behind you to lengthen the spine.

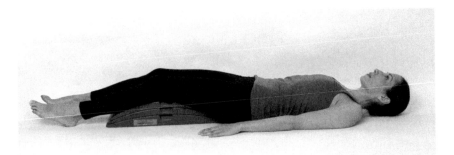

## 3. SIDE LYING STRETCH

Lie on your side and stretch over the Backbridge™. The highest point of the Backbridge™ should be at your rib cage. With your bottom hand, grab the wrist of your top hand and extend your arms overhead along the ground. Arm variations, including one to open the chest, are pictured below. As you progress, add more levels of the Backbridge™ to increase the stretch.

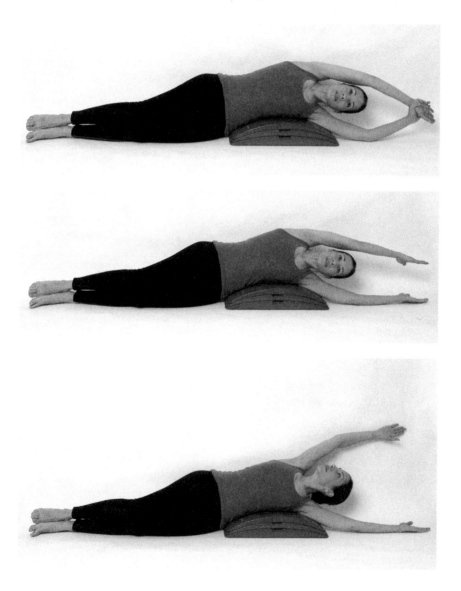

## 4. ABDOMINAL STRETCH (COBRA)

Lying face down over the Backbridge™, place your hands in front of you and do half a push-up so that your upper torso is elevated but your pelvis still has contact with the Backbridge™. Raise your eyes to the ceiling and hold for a count of five, then slowly lower yourself down and repeat. This stretch really works your lumbar extenders and lower back while stretching and lengthening the core (abdominals). The higher the level of the Backbridge™ you use, the easier the stretch will be.

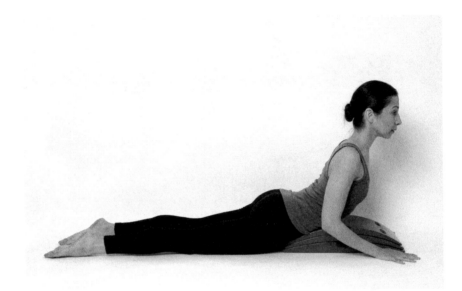

## 5. RECLINING TWIST

Place the Backbridge™ about 12 inches to the side of your hips. Keep your shoulders flat on the floor and bring one knee toward your chest. With the other leg flat on the floor, pull your bent knee over your torso, placing it on the Backbridge™. Hold the stretch and repeat on the opposite side. Try different levels of the Backbridge™ to find which is most comfortable for you (level 1 is the hardest.) It's important to keep both your shoulders on the mat during this stretch.

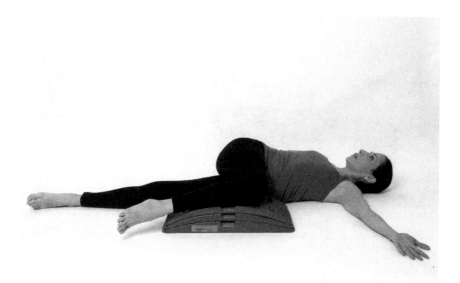

# 6. KNEES TO CHEST

Place your buttocks on the highest point of the Backbridge™ and lay back on the mat. Wrap your hands around your knees and gently pull your knees to your chest while reaching and lengthening your tailbone down toward the Backbridge™. Hold for a few seconds. If you have trouble wrapping your hands around your knees you can place them behind your legs. The higher the level you use in this posture, the more intense the stretch.

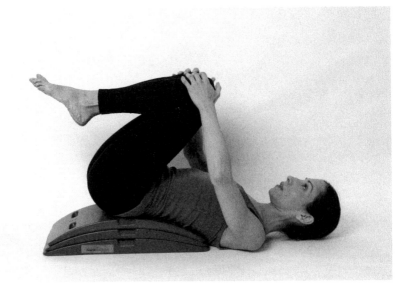

# 7. SINGLE KNEE TO CHEST

Pull one leg toward your chest and extend the opposite leg over the Back-bridge™ and along the mat. By gently angling the knee inward or outward, you will stretch different parts of your hip flexors.

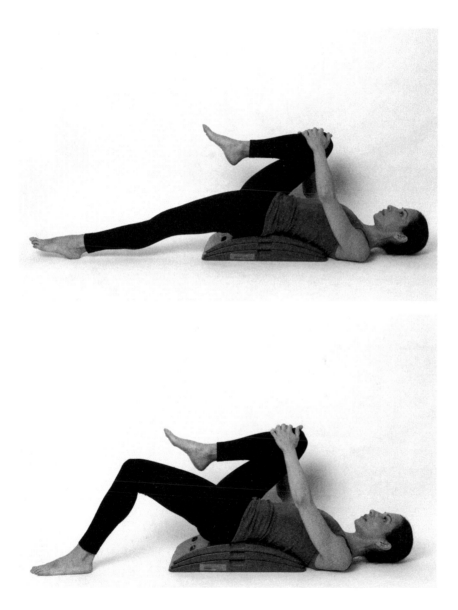

## 8. PIRIFORMIS AND OUTER HIP (FIGURE 4)

Place your buttocks on the highest point of the Backbridge™ and lie back on the floor. With both knees bent, cross one leg over the other, so that your legs form a number 4. Wrap your hands behind the uncrossed leg (or bottom knee) and gently pull toward you.

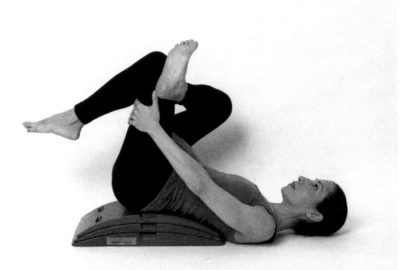

# 9. LOWER LATISSIMUS & LUMBAR ROTATORS

Sit on the top of the Backbridge™ and put your legs into a V position. Extend your right arm and place your right hand on your right ankle. Bring your left hand to meet your right and rotate your torso and head to face down, so that you are looking at your right knee. Hold this stretch then raise your left arm over your head and straighten it with the palm down, parallel to the floor. Breathe here, and lastly, look toward the ceiling to open the chest.

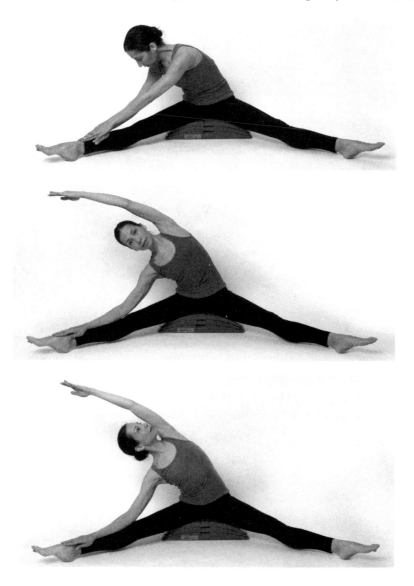

## 10. SEATED FORWARD FOLD

Sitting on the Backbridge™ as pictured, extend your legs out straight in front of you. Sit tall and fold at the hips, slowly bending forward over your legs as you reach toward your feet.

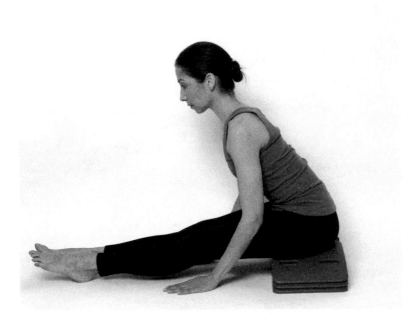

Investing in a Backbridge™ and integrating this quick routine into your day will help bring relief to your back pain within three weeks. On an ongoing basis, you will continue to surprise yourself as your flexibility and back vitality improve while you're aging.

# 7

# WHO TO SEE
# FOR STRUCTURAL SOLUTIONS

Each year, we spend more and more money on back pain treatments. It is estimated that Americans spend upwards of $80 billion a year. That is billions with a B! You probably think that the more resources spent on solving a problem, the better your results. Unfortunately, this is not the case. When it comes to back pain, who you see is what you get—which is why our current treatments for back pain haven't been working.

I cannot think of any other health issue where this is the case. If you are having a skin issue, you will see a dermatologist; a bunion, a podiatrist; a heart problem, a cardiologist. However, who will you see when you are suffering from a back problem? Will you see an orthopedist, neurologist, chiropractor, physical therapist, your primary care doctor, physiatrist, pain management specialist, orthopedic surgeon, massage therapist, or acupuncturist? Each of these specialties represent a unique perspective, training, and treatments. Unfortunately your treatment for back pain is not predicated on the cause of the true problem but rather which office you wind up in. A primary care doctor will prescribe medications, a physical therapist will prescribe exercise, a chiropractor will prescribe manipulation, and a surgeon will unfortunately recommend surgery. I believe that all of these specialists have your best interests at heart, but the confusion over who is the appropriate person to see is at the center of the back pain epidemic in this country.

While I have advocated self-treatment throughout this book, there are times when seeing the appropriate doctors at the right times is an important part of your treatment. My personal mantra is, "Start with the least invasive treatment and proceed from there."

My first recommendation is that you should always go for a yearly physical. Back pain can be a sign of some serious medical conditions; an annual check-up is always a good way to diagnose these types of problems as early as possible. There have been too many cases of patients ignoring low back pain for too long only to find out the back pain was something more serious, such as cancer. Your primary care doctor is well trained in diagnosing any serious medical condition and/or infection and is a good "rule out" person. On the other hand, general practitioners are usually not good "rule in" people because they receive only limited training in diagnosing and treating musculoskeletal conditions such as back pain.

If you have determined that your back pain is structural by using the Back Pain Inflammatory Index and after doing the recommended exercises in the book, you feel that you still need some professional help, here is a road map of "rule in" doctors to visit. Each level increases the amount of intervention and the risk, so start small in conjunction with your self-treatment plan and proceed only as necessary.

**Level 1:** chiropractor, physical therapist, or massage therapist

**Level 2:** non-surgical orthopedist (physiatrist) or internist

**Level 3:** orthopedist or neurologist

Level 1 practitioners are trained in the structure of your back and are experts in the musculoskeletal system. For example, a chiropractor will help realign your spine and a physical therapist will rehabilitate an injury. These things can work alongside your own efforts to improve your posture and counteract overuse, over-exercise or too much forward flexion in your day. A massage therapist can loosen the tight muscular system, but the therapist shouldn't be the first or only doctor you visit, because muscular tension often comes from an unbalanced spine. Trying to massage a muscle that is not in balance will not only fail to balance the muscle but will cause greater irritation and inflammation. But a combination of a chiropractor and a massage therapist might be the best way to restore balance and release the muscles that have been tense due to that imbalance.

Testing by Level 1 practitioners may include spinal X rays, bloodwork, urinalysis, computerized range of motion and strength testing. Within three weeks under active care from a Level 1 provider, you really should notice significant improvements.

If you don't feel a response to your Level 1 practitioners in three to four weeks, go back to the beginning and make sure that you're first identifying the correct cause of your pain and secondly that your practitioner is open to and properly treating that cause. If both of these things seem to be true, advance to a Level 2 provider. Chiropractors and physical therapists are trained to evaluate if the patient may need to see a Level 2 or 3 practitioner, so the hope is that they will guide you toward an experienced and reputable physician. Level 2 internists are good at ruling out any significant problems, as well as prescribing pain medications that may be necessary at this point for a patient. Non-surgical orthopedists, called physiatrists, are MDs trained in physical medicine and rehabilitation. Their training and perspective is based on NON-surgical methods, which according to our "least-to-most" approach on the invasive scale, is best. They are quite adept at diagnosis and have a strong understanding of medications and different types of injections that may help you until your body heals from the cause of its pain. Testing by Level 2 practitioners might include nerve conduction test, more detailed physical, neurologist consults, trigger point injections, or steroid blocks.

Neurologists and orthopedic surgeons comprise Level 3. This level comes with the greatest level of risk and intervention. If you have eliminated the possibility that your symptoms could be caused by nutritional and emotional factors, you should be consulting these type of practitioners. I have seen numerous patients, who have previously had spine surgery with little improvement, achieve excellent results after determining the exact cause of their pain with the Back Pain Inflammatory Index!

## THE THREE-WEEK TAKE-AWAY

### Three Easy Tips to Help You Target Your Structural Solution

The tips in this section are designed to help you fix the little things. And fixing little things can make a big difference.

### *1. Extension, extension, extension.*

Most of us are doing too much sitting or other activities that cause forward hunching, thereby creating a C-shaped posture in our body. Combat your core imbalance by laying over a Backbridge™, yoga ball, or rolled up towel for two minutes twice a day, or at the very least, incorporate extension and release stretches, like the Standing Abdominal stretch or Thumbs to Pits stretch, so that you can regain proper posture!

### *2. Move and stretch!*

Our daily lives have become too sedentary, particularly for the average office worker. Get up throughout your day, even if it's just to go to the copy machine or stand up and stretch while you take a call. You should also find time to move aerobically three times a week for thirty minutes. Walking is one of my favorite exercises for back pain sufferers. It stimulates the entire body, gets the blood flowing, and allows you to clear your head. Studies have shown that music is a great relaxer so put on headphones, get into your groove and start walking.

### *3. Don't look down!*

When texting or looking at your phone or tablet, keep your head up! Lowering your head puts tremendous pressure on your neck and shoulders (10 pounds for every 10 degrees your head is bent). Looking straight ahead can save you LOADS of neck pain!

# Nutritional Diagnosis and Solutions

# 8

# DIGESTIVE EVALUATION

The world of digestive upsets is not a welcoming one. You may be aware that you have a sensitive stomach, but you may not realize how far-reaching the chemical effects have on the rest of your body. In fact, the most overlooked cause of back pain is diet. While there are thousands of studies on how nutrition impacts muscular function, very few health professionals have connected the dots from back pain to digestive function and nutrition. Poor digestive function will elevate your inflammatory factor, thus creating more back pain.

If the Back Pain Inflammatory Index has revealed that you have back pain stemming from a digestive or chemical cause, you are not alone. In one study published by the *Asian Spine Journal* in 2014, 31% of women and 24.6% of men who were suffering from back pain also suffered from gastrointestinal (GI) complaints such as abdominal pain or food intolerance. My patient, Jon, is a prime example of how diet can both cause and compound back pain.

•   •   •

I HAVE SOMETHING *called degenerative disc disease and have had a poor back for the best part of ten years. The key thing about my condition is that the problem is at many levels (T9 through L4), not just in one segment of the back. In 2010, I had a major surgery in London, where I lived at the time, which resulted in the insertion of two titanium rods and 14 screws from T9 through L4, as well as the fusion of a couple of vertebrae from T11 to L1. After struggling with the metal, I had the surgery reversed and the rods and screws removed in 2012.*

*Around that time, I moved to the United States for work and discovered Dr. Sinett. He sat me down and spoke about his unique approach. Dr. Sinett then did some very strange maneuvers in his office, lifting my arms and legs and such. He talked about structural care but specifically honed in on my diet. I'm in okay shape, I exercise, and I didn't think I ate too poorly. But he wanted more than that. He rubbed my gut and told me that my stomach was inflamed and irritated. I had no idea it was irritated! He then talked about toxicity and his diet for back pain. I told my friends and they thought it was strange—some of the things I was permitted to eat on the diet, like nuts, were high in calories! Dr. Sinett's diet had a totally different approach. It was not a weight loss diet, but a diet to reduce my gut inflammation. Nuts, as he explained, are low in toxins, so they were on his "Yes" list.*

*It took me six months to buy into Dr. Sinett's nutrition plan. For that time, I'd do the diet for three days, then the weekend came, and I'd forget it. It was so unique compared to anything I had seen or witnessed, I just wasn't convinced—and after living in London and Dubai, I had seen a whole host of doctors and experienced many different facets of international healthcare! But with Dr. Sinett, you can't cheat, because if you go in there for a few weeks and say you have been doing the diet, he can just feel your gut and other points on your body and tell pretty quickly that you haven't! Ultimately, I was kidding myself.*

*Finally, I committed to the diet for a month, which led to two months because I noticed marked improvement in my pain. On his diet, you don't go hungry! You can eat plenty of food and it isn't complex to follow— there is just a list of things to avoid. Even though the diet isn't calorie controlled, after a few months, I surprisingly lost 24 pounds. I felt a lot better because I wasn't bloated or sore—I wasn't even aware I was bloated or sore until I no longer had that feeling! I learned if your gut is upset, pain can radiate around to your back. So the diet is massive, and for me, it's been very helpful when it seemed little else was helping.*

*Now, I follow Dr. Sinett's diet, I work to keep my emotions in check, and I meet with the physical therapist in his office to keep myself in structural health, which is complementary, and there aren't many facilities that I've found that offer that set-up. If I go out of sync on one of those three things, I fall down. I've just had a great Christmas, for example, but a rubbish Christmas from my diet perspective, and I know I have to knuckle back on it, because I have the confidence now that getting on track will keep my back up to par. I can manage my process a lot better by having met Dr. Sinett.*

*From a surgical perspective, my major operation was technically perfect. It just didn't help me. Dr. Sinett could have helped without having the surgery at all, and anyone with back pain facing surgery should certainly see Dr. Sinett as a matter of course.*

*Jon Mann*

## WE ARE WHAT WE EAT

Our bodies and back will only function as well as the fuel we put into them (input), and how we eliminate our waste material (output). Let's start at the beginning with the input. The fuel you put into your body is what can throw your GI system—and your back—totally off (as can stress or hormones, which will be discussed later). In my practice, I have treated people who suffer from back pain because they drink too much coffee or alcohol and eat too much sugar. But healthy foods can also be the culprit. Some people have back pain from eating too much salad!

If you've ever had a hangover, you can guess how the whole thing works. Our bodies react to what we eat with a viscero-somatic response. *Viscero* means "organ"; *somatic* refers to your body—in this case, the musculoskeletal system. Some of what we consume is soothing to our body; some irritates and causes pain. This viscero-somatic response to what we eat can range from being alert after your morning coffee, to feeling sleepy from the tryptophan in turkey, to getting an upset stomach from something acidic, to developing back pain. Consuming a large quantity of inflammatory foods may cause your muscles to contract without relaxing. If this goes on for a prolonged period of time, back spasms and other negative health issues will result.

Caffeine, alcohol, and sugar are part of many people's daily diets and these substances have been shown to increase cortisol levels. Cortisol is a chemical produced by the body during stressful situations. When too much is present in a body, connective tissue throughout the body can become inflamed, causing pain. Other poor eating habits such as consuming very large meals, skipping meals, or consuming only low-carb foods can result in low blood sugar and create more stress in the body. Chronically elevated cortisol levels increase your appetite and cravings for calorie-dense sweets and salty snacks, so the negative cycle continues. All of these factors can ultimately trigger an inflammatory reaction that results in back pain.

Some foods are known to be inflammatory while others are anti-inflammatory. Eating right counteracts the inflammatory process in the body. To find the underlying chemical cause of pain, the first step is to determine whether there have been changes in your eating pattern that would alter the chemical system, or whether you have developed a repetitive eating pattern that has become toxic and, over time, has broken down the body's natural resistance. This may include eating too much of a "good thing," such as raw fruits and vegetables and other roughage. As we determine the right nutrition solution for you, you'll want to think about your pain pattern and see if you can trace your pain to poor dietary choices that also result in reflux, gas pains, diarrhea, or constipation. Proper foods for your system will be the best medicine you can get!

## The Scoop on Poop

Before we tackle your specific nutrition sensitivities, let's address output. Output has been largely ignored and is just as important as, if not more so, than what you are putting into your body. Yes, the quality of your bowel movements absolutely relates to quality of your back! It tells us what is going on in your digestive process—and directly correlates to how your nutrients affect you.

One of the most common but missed causes of back pain is improper bowel movements, i.e., constipation and diarrhea. When people suffer from constipation their body builds up with toxicity. Waste material that should be exiting the body winds up not exiting in a timely manner. Once this toxicity builds, it impacts your muscular system by elevating the inflammation factor. Diarrhea can result in the same type of inflammatory reaction from the body; only with diarrhea, the intestinal system is unable to properly process waste material and excretes it too soon, irritating the intestinal system. An irritated digestive and intestinal system can then affect the muscular system. In short, what you put in must be able to be processed effectively by your digestive system and excreted in a healthy, consistent way.

Normal bowel habits do vary. When we talk about regularity, what we're really talking about is *what's regular for you*. Three bowel movements per day to three per week is considered the normal range.

What's more important than frequency is the ease with which you move your bowels. If you need to push or strain, something is off. Many factors can affect regularity, such as diet, travel, medications, hormonal fluctuations, sleep patterns, exercise, and stress. The characteristics of your stool (the color, odor, shape, size) will tell you a good deal about how happy and healthy your digestive tract is.

So, let's look at the toilet bowl! The Bristol Stool Chart is a handy tool that may help you learn what you're going for. Ideally, your stool should approximate Types 3, 4 and 5, "like a sausage or a snake, smooth and soft" to "soft blobs that pass easily." Type 4 is the ideal. If you regularly see these types of stools, your input is working for your system and being properly eliminated.

## BRISTOL STOOL CHART

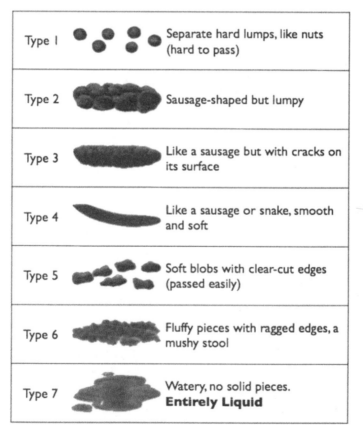

| Type 1 | | Separate hard lumps, like nuts (hard to pass) |
| --- | --- | --- |
| Type 2 | | Sausage-shaped but lumpy |
| Type 3 | | Like a sausage but with cracks on its surface |
| Type 4 | | Like a sausage or snake, smooth and soft |
| Type 5 | | Soft blobs with clear-cut edges (passed easily) |
| Type 6 | | Fluffy pieces with ragged edges, a mushy stool |
| Type 7 | | Watery, no solid pieces. **Entirely Liquid** |

*Reproduced with kind permission of Dr KW Heaton, formerly Reader in Medicine at the University of Bristol. ©2000, Norgine group of companies.*

▶ **TIP: GET YOUR GI ON TRACK!** If you become constipated, increase your water intake, eat fruits, vegetables and other high-fiber foods, and exercise to stimulate the bowels. If you are having diarrhea, decrease your fiber intake and participate in a stress-reducing activity. If diarrhea is a recurring problem, consider food sensitivities or allergies and pay attention to how your bowels change after consuming certain foods. A simple way to keep your GI tract on track is to drink a tall glass of cold water. This should help get your digestive and elimination systems jump started.

Of course, these are fixes for the occasional bout of an upset stomach. Back pain that is induced by digestive causes requires a change in your nutrition in order to affect your output and eliminate back pain. A happy digestive system is the key for a good feeling back!

So what foods should we input to create optimal digestion and healthy output? The following chapters will explain the food rules for a healthy back and give you dietary options based on the specific digestive cause of your back pain!

## CURIOUS ABOUT COLONICS?

People frequently ask me my opinion on colonics. I have personally never had one but have had patients who have gotten great relief from them. My recommendation would be to use them as a last resort after you have tried to balance out both the output and input aspects of your digestive system. Colonics are great to clean you out, but ideally you want to get to the cause of your discomfort or pain.

# THE SAVVY SHOPPER'S CHEAT SHEET FOR BUYING ORGANIC

More and more people are buying organic food because it tastes better and is free of pesticides and other chemicals. A recent study has found that organic strawberries, and blackberries have up to 50% more antioxidants—chemicals that fight illnesses such as cancer and heart disease. I encourage you to include as many organic products in your No More Back Pain Diet as you can. In addition, you can also look for grass-fed, free-range meats. I know organic foods often come with a higher price tag and are not always readily available so it may not be practical for you to buy all organic for the three-week duration of the diet, and for years after as you adhere to this diet.

## What should you splurge on and on what items can you save?

The Environmental Working Group (EWG) has identified what it calls The Dirty Dozen Plus™, or the fruits and veggies with the most pesticide residues. You can lower your pesticide intake by choosing organic for these foods:

| | |
|---|---|
| Apples | Peaches |
| Celery | Potatoes |
| Cherry Tomatoes | Spinach |
| Cucumbers | Strawberries |
| Grapes | Sweet Bell Peppers |
| Hot Peppers | Kale/Collard Greens |
| Imported Nectarines | Summer Squash |

The EWG's "Clean Fifteen™" include fruits and vegetables with the least pesticide residue, so these are foods that are safe to skip in the organic aisle and buy in the regular produce section:

| | |
|---|---|
| Asparagus | Mangos |
| Avocados | Mushrooms |
| Cabbage | Onions |
| Cantaloupe | Papaya |
| Sweet Corn | Pineapples |
| Eggplant | Sweet Peas—Frozen |
| Grapefruit | Sweet Potatoes |
| Kiwi | |

## *If buying organic is not an option*

If you don't have the option to buy organic, be sure to properly wash all of your fruits and vegetables before you eat them!

# STARTING SIMPLE:
# BASIC FOOD RULES FOR A HEALTHY BACK

One Saturday afternoon, I received a call from a Grammy-winning recording artist who was suffering from severe upper back and neck pain and was concerned that she wasn't going to be able to make it through her performance on *Saturday Night Live* and a concert that was scheduled for the following day. She said the pain was so bad that she could barely turn her head.

I examined her and noticed her whole muscular system was tight, almost to the point of rigidity, as if she was suffering from a full-body spasm. I also could tell she was suffering from severe gas pains, and she revealed to me that her on-the-road diet was primarily fast-food and processed foods. I immediately knew the root of her problem.

The good news was we had a diagnosis—back pain stemming from an inflamed digestive system, and a solution—a healthy nutrition plan. The bad news was I couldn't cure her immediately. When a physical reaction is that severe, it reflects a toxic buildup within the body, which requires a reorientation of the diet and time for the body to readjust.

I've seen many cases like this, especially when patients say they don't have much time to prepare meals. The average daily food log I review looks something like this:

**Breakfast:** coffee, muffin or bagel, more coffee

**Lunch:** sandwich, chips, soda or iced tea

**Snack:** candy or chips, soda or coffee

**Dinner:** pizza or pasta, soda or wine, pastry or ice cream

Your body is a high-performance engine, and filling it with low-performance fuels doesn't provide enough of the vitamins and nutrients you need to function. Consuming foods described above leave you with energy crashes and irritate the delicate balance of your digestive system, sending pain right through to your back.

On the flip side, about 20 percent of patients I encounter describe themselves as "health nuts." Fruits and vegetables, including big raw salads, smoothies, and other roughage, are the foundation of their diet. They also suffer from back pain induced by digestive issues. These people are eating too many "healthy" foods. The lack of variety in their diet and the over-consumption of one or two food groups irritates their digestive systems. These patients complain of gassiness, bloating, abdominal pain, diarrhea, and even constipation. Ultimately, the body needs multiple sources of vitamins, minerals, and other nutrients. When it comes to the body, balance and variety is key. By introducing whole grains, more protein, and even some dairy, the transit time becomes more accommodating for positive absorption and back pain goes away.

Before I understood this, I went on my own health kick. I started having high-fiber oatmeal every day for breakfast and a salad for lunch. A week into this diet, I had a dramatic increase in bloating and stomach pain—and eventually a stiff neck. When I returned to my old eating habits, which were already pretty healthy, I felt better. The moral of the story is this: Just because a food is healthy doesn't mean it is always good for you—or something you should eat every day.

Here are some healthy foods that cause trouble when eaten repetitively:

| | |
|---|---|
| Salad | Raw Vegetables |
| Oatmeal | Frozen Yogurt |
| Egg Whites | Beans |
| Tofu | Fresh-squeezed juices |
| Smoothies | Protein Bars |

Too much roughage is the biggest culprit, since it causes your digestive tract to go into overdrive. This can happen very quickly and cause an immediate spike in back pain, just like it did for Heidi. Here's her story:

•  •  •

MY NAME IS *Heidi Krupp, and I am the last person who should be writing a testimonial. The reason being, for full disclosure, that Dr. Sinett hired me to do PR for this book. After meeting Dr. Sinett and looking over his manuscript in my office, I thought he had a great concept and a* worthy book. His whole-body integrative approach, which we call "The Sinett Solution," seemed different than all the other back pain books before it. I was convinced I "got it" and went about to create a marketing and PR plan to promote 3 Weeks to a Better Back.

In the beginning of 2015, I decided to kickstart my health and started a raw diet to cleanse and shed those 10 extra pounds. I was simultaneously running a PR campaign for a well-known book author, which, while exciting, had me flying all over the country. Right after the campaign ended, I decided to go to south Florida for some well-deserved rest. While my back always bothered me a bit, I generally didn't pay much attention and with the right angling of my body getting up, and avoiding lifting heavy things, I could get through the day and "manage." This all changed for me on the flight back from Florida when my back pain unexpectedly and ferociously became completely unmanageable. My back was crooked, I could barely walk and the amount of pain that I was in rivaled childbirth with my son. I was downright scared and convinced that I had blown out a disc in my lower back. I reached out to Dr. Sinett, who told me to come into his office the next morning.

We started the examination by talking. Dr. Sinett listened to me describe my back pain, which was now radiating down my left hip and parts of my leg, as well as my concern of a herniating disc. I asked him about an immediate MRI to figure this out. Dr. Sinett told me that while a disc herniation was a possibility, it wasn't likely, and reminded me of what I had read in his manuscript: that the only random thing in the body is trauma, such as a fall or car accident, and everything else builds little by little. Like a detective, Dr. Sinett went back and asked me all sorts of questions about what I was doing before my back went out. Questions like, "How are your stress levels?" "Are you doing anything differently?" "Did you change your diet?" After telling him about my stress and my New Year's diet resolution, Dr. Sinett just smiled and started to examine me.

The examination started like ones that I have had before when my back was giving me a little trouble. But this time, just lying down on his table was an ordeal because the pain was so severe. Dr. Sinett tested my strength and flexibility, which were both poor. He then ran what he called orthopedic tests to help determine where my back pain was coming from. Finally, he pressed into my stomach by my right hip and it immediately killed. (Kidney stones, too? I thought.) He pushed into the rest of my stomach and explained that this was a buildup of gas, *probably caused by my new raw diet regimen. After pushing on these points, immediately my strength returned and I felt a little better. Dr. Sinett explained to me that anything that could upset your digestive system could create muscular spasms in your back. He surmised that the raw diet upset my digestive system, and he wanted me to change my diet for the next few days. No raw vegetables but rather soothing foods, as if I was getting over a stomach bug. I had chicken soup, a grilled cheese, broiled fish and even some toast, and I tried to find a little time to make for myself after my busy workday. I went back to see him for the next few days and my pain got less and less. In less than a week, I went from being unable to walk and tie my own shoes to feeling completely normal—even better than I had before my back was bothering me.*

*In looking back at this experience from Dr. Sinett, I learned some remarkable things; most importantly, that it wasn't my back. I agree that I had back pain but the cause wasn't a problem with my spine, but rather stress and diet. The other thing I learned was the concern for other back pain sufferers. What would have happened if I had not met Dr. Sinett and wound up having the typical treatments for back pain? I would have had an MRI, had some pain medication, done some stretches, and eventually the pain would have returned to a manageable level—most likely after I tired of my raw food diet and removed that inflammatory factor. I would have spent my life managing my mediocre back, and I would have had numerous episodes of this severe back pain because I would have never equated my fad diets and work stress to being the cause of my back pain.*

*Now after this back pain experience, I finally got it! Reading the manuscript wasn't enough for the truth to set in. I had to actually live it. Not only am I feeling tons better but this new understanding has completely changed my perspective on back pain and health forever. This book can make a world of difference for back pain sufferers. It certainly did for me!*

*Heidi Krupp*

## Quick Tips for Eating Well

- ▶ Eat something within one hour of getting up each morning.

- ▶ Have at least one healthful snack between meals each day.

- ▶ Eat slowly to allow yourself to be aware of feeling full.

▶ Avoid the clean-plate club. Always leave at least one bite of each type of food on your plate at the end of the meal.

▶ Keep a food journal.

## Hone In On the Issue

If you have nutritionally induced back pain, I highly recommend you start with an input/output journal to help you identify:

1. Where there is repetition in your diet and thus, where you lack variety
2. Which foods create certain feelings or digestive upsets (i.e., gassiness, bloating, diarrhea, constipation)
3. The time of your meals and snacks and amount you eat
4. Whether there are circumstances that affect your consumption and elimination, such as travel, illness, or special events.

Don't modify what you eat when you start the journal because the purpose of this written record is to evaluate your normal eating, drinking, and elimination patterns in order to identify the foods that may upset your system such as the usual suspects including too much sugar, processed foods, caffeine, alcohol, or roughage. Noting the time you consume your foods will show whether you are going too long between eating, eating too much, or eating too little.

# FOOD RULES FOR HEALTHY BACKS

I have seven simple rules to help patients maintain a healthy back.

## 1. Watch your weight

Being overweight is a contributing factor to structural imbalance. The more you weigh, the more your bones and naturally, your spine must bear. However, excess weight is a greater factor in back problems because of the toxicity and unhealthy eating habits that trigger inflammation. While extra pounds do cause structural pain, it's what's happening on the inside that is more likely to be causing your pain.

## 2. Drink plenty of water

Many of my patients simply don't drink enough water. Coffee, iced tea, and beer do not constitute fluid and actually dehydrate you. Lack of water causes the area around the spinal discs to become dry, and little fissures, or cracks, can form. If the fissures become severe, then the inside of the discs can bulge and put pressure on your spinal nerves or spinal cord. Staying hydrated with plain, pure water can help prevent this painful condition.

## 3. Cut down on caffeine

Caffeine increases muscle contractions, which means that those back cramps or spasms could be caused by your daily cup of Joe, especially if you find yourself consuming it in large doses.

## 4. Count on calcium

Calcium helps us fight off arthritis and osteoarthritis, two causes of debilitating pain. When it comes to calcium, you need to consider not just the amount of calcium that you consume (or take in supplement form), but the amount that your body is able to absorb. It's important to get Vitamin D (through sun or supplements), which helps the body absorb calcium, but it's also vital that you change lifestyles that block absorption.

In 1993, a group of Yale University researchers studied the occurrence of hip fractures in 16 countries; they expected the countries that had a population with the greatest calcium consumption would have the fewest hip fractures. Surprisingly, the countries where people had high calcium intake actually had more hip fractures! That's because the population in these countries also had high consumption of processed foods, caffeine, alcohol, sugar, sodium, and tobacco, all of which deplete calcium from the body and increase the chances of bone breaks and arthritic pain.

## 5. So long, sweeteners!

The average American consumes some 175 pounds of sugar each year— including about 600 cans of soda a year, at ten teaspoons of sugar or the equivalent of artificial sweetener a pop. Too much sugar not only increases the rate at which you excrete calcium, but it also can irritate the digestive system and cause back pain.

## 6. Beware of any word that ends in -ose

Start reading your food labels. You'll probably find that much of what you consume includes substances with names you probably can't pronounce. Food is primarily made up of the first four or five ingredients listed on the label so pay attention to the order in which the ingredients are listed. Ingredients ending in -ose are sugars, and prepared foods and condiments are loaded with them. Watch out for these other red-flag ingredients:

1. Hydrogenated or partially hydrogenated oils.
2. Trans-fats, which are made when vegetable oils are exposed to hydrogen so that they solidify at room temperature. Trans-fats were added to foods because they lengthen shelf life; unfortunately, they are detrimental to our health and are now being removed from many foods.
3. Interesterified fat, called interesterified soybean or stated rich oil on food labels, has been shown to lower HDL, or good, cholesterol, increase blood glucose levels, and depress insulin.
4. Enriched wheat flour, which is neither whole wheat nor oat bran flour and does not deliver the nutrients and fiber you need.
5. Other additives, including those that end with -ates or -ites, like nitrates and nitrites, which are found in processed meats.
6. Food coloring, because it's an unnatural ingredient!
7. Tyramine, a naturally occurring substance formed from the breakdown of protein as food ages. It's found in alcoholic beverages, aged cheeses, and processed meats and has been associated with increased systolic blood pressure and migraines.

## The most important rule is #7: Listen to your body

Just because your taste buds like something doesn't mean your stomach does. Your body knows what is good for it and what isn't—you just have to listen and obey. If you had Chinese food last night and you don't feel well this morning, ask yourself whether it was the three beers you had with dinner or the food itself. If you routinely get a stomachache after consuming milk products, you might have lactose intolerance. If you really pay attention to your body's signals, you can avoid the foods that upset your system and find both relief in your stomach and your back! The No More Back Pain Diet will help you formulate a balanced eating plan and help you tap into the messages your body is sending you.

# 9

# THE NO MORE BACK PAIN DIET

N ow we know diet has a huge impact on back pain. Muscles and organs contract and relax in the process of doing their jobs. Their motions make digestion possible, but refined carbohydrates, excess sugar, and caffeine throw our stomachs into turmoil and cause the muscles involved in digestion to contract for an extended period. The result? Spasms and pain.

If you racked up more than five points in the digestive evaluation of the Back Pain Inflammatory Test, choosing a healthful, balanced diet will help you input the right things into your body, digest properly, and eliminate efficiently, thus reducing the chemical inflammation that is causing your back pain and preventing it from recurring. The "No More Back Pain" Diet has been designed to target and eliminate certain toxins from your system. It will make a dramatic difference in the way your body functions and how you feel, both in your back and throughout the rest of your body.

The No More Back Pain Diet works for about 80% of those suffering from digestive-induced back pain (Don't worry, if you are in the other 20%, I will explain alternate plans that are tailored to suit your needs). The No More Back Pain Diet addresses different levels of pain (from mild to severe) and offers various starting points, depending on the severity of your pain. The Diet for Severe Back Pain is for people who can barely move. If you have trouble getting out of bed and can't bend to tie your shoes, you should start with this plan, follow it for four days and then transition into the Mild to Moderate plan, which is the plan sufferers with lesser pain will start on. The No More Back Pain Diet includes easy long-term maintenance support that will enable you to successfully stick to it.

The problem with other diets is that they take a one-size-fits-all approach and each person has individual needs that must be met to work with his or her chemical balance. The No More Back Pain Diet can be tailored to your tastes. As you start to follow this new diet plan, listen to your body. How do you feel after you start the diet? The ideal eating plan leaves you feeling satisfied and energized. If you feel gassy, bloated, or fatigued after a meal, you didn't eat the right foods. So, over the course of the next three weeks, follow the plan, listen to the signals of your digestive system and carefully monitor changes in your back pain. Weaning yourself from the foods that create inflammation and replacing them with foods that your system can properly process will produce relief from pain in just three weeks.

- - -

I STARTED EXPERIENCING *back pain in the late 90s after participating in a 'hora' at a friend's wedding. After months of doctor visits, pain pills, and physical therapy, my pain finally subsided, but I always felt like it would reappear. I walked cautiously and gingerly in an effort not to reactivate it. As a rather fit 37-year-old, I was depressed thinking I would have this condition for the rest of my life. My Uncle Frank had a bad back and was in constant pain and discomfort; this was not something I desired!*

*In 2001, I started a new job and a colleague named Phil noticed I had discomfort when sitting and standing. He mentioned a chiropractor/ kinesiologist, Dr. Sinett, whom he had been going to with great success. Eliminate my back pain? I was game!*

*I made an appointment and went to see Dr. Sinett. Phil had cautioned me that this would not be a typical doctor's visit . . . and boy, was he right! Immediately, what struck me was how nice everyone in the office was. I was led into a room where I met Dr. Sinett; after asking me a few questions about my symptoms, general health, exercise routines, and diet, he made a particularly unusual request: to take my shoes off and stand on a pencil! As I did this, he pushed down on my arm. Sometimes my arm could barely resist the force and other times I could resist. Phil* was right . . . this was not like any other doctor's visit! Dr. Sinett then asked me questions while having me place my hand on my head. Finally, the doctor concluded that my back pain was not the result of structural issues but was primarily due to stress and a poor diet.

Yes, I had a stressful job in finance, and I could see how that might affect my back, but I did not see the correlation to my diet, which was poor at best.

Dr. Sinett recommended that I reduce the processed food in my diet and start a cleanse as a way to flush out and detox my system. I followed his recommendation and within a week started seeing results. Not only did my back pain go away, but my digestion was much better, my weight started dropping, my mood was lighter, and I felt less stress. My body, muscles, and tendons all felt looser.

I have been under Dr. Sinett's care for more than 12 years now. Combining an improved diet and daily use of the Backbridge™ has virtually eliminated my back discomfort. Now I am not perfect, and sometimes I am not as careful with my diet as I should be. When I feel my body becoming less flexible, it's my sign to get back on my diet. I always get great results!

I no longer live in the New York City area. In 2011, I moved my home to the Poconos in Pennsylvania, where I work as a personal and business results coach and serve as a seasonal park ranger with the National Park Service. I've tried other chiropractors in my area, spent a lot of money and invested lots of time to be told I have to come back twice a week for months to 'fix' and maintain the structural problems with my back. I NEVER got the results I get with Dr. Sinett and currently make the three-state trek just to see him. It's the only way to treat my spine, as well as my well-being.

John Beljean

# THE DIET

## Approved Foods

▶ Whole grains, including whole grain breads, pastas, cereals, tortillas, and baked goods (look for the words whole grain on the food label followed by the name of the grain, such as wheat, corn, rice, oats, barley, quinoa, sorghum, and rye)

- Oatmeal or Cornmeal

- Soy Flour

- Nuts and seeds, including nut and seed oils, nut and seed butters, unsweetened coconut, vegetable oils, olive oil, and flaxseed oil

- Protein, including chicken, fish (especially mackerel, lake trout, herring, sardines, albacore tuna, and salmon), lean cuts of meat (turkey, pork, beef), eggs, and cheese

- Vegetables, all including starchy vegetables such as sweet potatoes, potatoes, corn, butternut squash, and peas

- Fruit, all except those listed on the non-approved list

- Decaffeinated coffee and tea (unsweetened)

- Seltzer water, plain and flavored (but the only ingredients should be water and natural flavor)

- Water

## Non-Approved Foods

- Enriched white flour, commonly found in breads, pasta, biscuits, waffles, crackers, muffins, cereal, pancakes, croutons, rolls, pretzels, graham crackers, cookies, baked goods, and tortillas

- Hydrogenated oils (look for the words trans-fat, partially hydrogenated oil, and hydrogenated oil on the food label)*

- Cream cheese and processed cheeses

- Some fruits, such as grapes, bananas, cherries, figs, and dried fruit

- Artificially flavored and/or sweetened fruit drinks*

- Grape Juice (even unsweetened)

- Milk shakes and malts

- Soft drinks, including diet sodas*

- Meal-replacement shakes

- Hot chocolate and chocolate milk

▶ Wine, beer, spirits, and cordials

▶ Caffeinated coffee and tea

▶ Added sweeteners, including sugar, molasses, honey, agave, nectar, and artificial sweeteners

▶ Packaged or processed food (look for words ending in -ose on the food label)

Some of the non-approved foods can be added to your diet once you have completed three weeks of Phase 2. You should always try to avoid the foods marked with an asterisk (*) even when you've reached the maintenance phase.

## GETTING STARTED

Plan to begin this diet on a Friday. Over the weekend, you're more likely to have a flexible schedule so you won't be too inconvenienced if you suffer from caffeine and sugar withdrawal.

### Shopping

Get rid of the junk food in your house and stock up on healthy, approved foods. Initially, this diet may be more expensive than the foods that you've been consuming, but once you purchase the basics, healthy eating generally costs about the same as consuming prepackaged junk food. And, your continued health is certainly worth any extra cost!

### Cook Ahead

Prep for the week ahead over the weekend. Create a meal and snack plan and prepare foods that you can eat throughout the week such as grilled chicken, boiled eggs, fresh cut-up veggies, and small baggies of nuts. Once you establish this routine, it will be easy to keep going.

## Don't Let Yourself Get Too Hungry

The recommended portion sizes are guidelines, but you may need to adjust them to meet your needs. Remember, this is not a weight loss diet, though many people will lose weight when they're on it. Getting too hungry will likely cause you to overeat, so it's better to include snacks to insure that you don't overindulge or binge.

## Commit to Three Weeks

You should maintain this diet for three weeks; that is how long it will take your body to feel chemically different and for you to establish a new habit. It is okay if you make a few missteps but you should just get right back to the diet. Don't sabotage yourself further just because you had a cookie in the conference room! Too many people use one slip-up as a diet deal breaker. One cookie won't make you fat and one cookie won't cause tremendous back pain. However, if you follow up that cookie with a soda, another cookie, and so on and so forth, you will be back to square one. Commit to three full weeks of this new eating plan, and after that, you'll find yourself gravitating toward the healthy foods and you'll be less likely to fall back into old, unhealthy habits.

# PHASE 1: DIET FOR SEVERE BACK PAIN

When you're suffering from severe back pain, your body is dealing with inflammation. Before you can feel the benefits of removing toxins and irritants from your diet, you must let your muscles and digestive system calm down. The goal of this phase of the diet is to remove inflammation. Just as you can easily survive for a few days of only eating soup and toast when you have a stomach bug, it is also acceptable for you to eat only the foods on this bland diet for a few days.

### Basic Action

Although it may counter all of the diet advice you've heard, you're going to remove all of the fiber, or roughage, from your diet. This means you cannot eat any whole grains, nuts, or raw fruits, and vegetables. However, you may eat them well-cooked! Roughage is, well, rough to digest and while it will be added back in for Phase 2, you first need to clear your system. You must also cut out chips, spicy food, caffeine and alcohol. This is the Clean Slate Phase, designed to create a calm environment within your body that is receptive to the healthful and nutritious changes you'll make in the next phase, The Mild to ModeratePlan.

This "clean slate" phase is filled with easily digestible carbohydrates, which, although limited in nutritional content, are virtually fiber-free and are easy to process. Foods like white rice and white bread give the system time to heal, and once your inflammation has calmed down, you'll switch to multi-grains.

### Duration

Follow this phase for three to four days if you regularly drink caffeine or alcohol. One or two days may be enough for people who don't usually drink these beverages.

### What to Expect

This diet will feel a little boring, but fortunately, you only follow it for a few days. If you are a big coffee or soda drinker, you will probably go through caffeine withdrawal, leading to flu-like symptoms or headaches which may last almost a week. If you are accustomed to high-fiber cereal, fruits, and veggies, you may feel deprived and could experience mild constipation.

# Sample Meals

**DAY 1**

■ BREAKFAST

4 ounces fruit juice (not grape)

1 cup puffed rice cereal with skim or unsweetened soy milk

6 ounces plain non- or low-fat yogurt with cinnamon

1 cup decaffeinated herbal tea

■ LUNCH

1 grilled cheese sandwich on white bread

1 cup of chicken noodle soup

■ DINNER

Mixed steamed vegetables with a little butter or margarine

1 grilled or broiled filet mignon

1 baked potato without skin, topped with plain yogurt and chives

**DAY 2**

■ BREAKFAST

4 ounces fruit juice (not grape)

2 scrambled eggs

2 pieces white toast with butter

1 cup decaf herbal tea

■ LUNCH

1 grilled chicken breast on a roll with mayonnaise

■ DINNER

1½ cups roast chicken

Roasted potatoes, equivalent to one potato

Well-cooked peas, broccoli, or green beans

## DAY 3

■ BREAKFAST

4 ounces fruit juice (not grape)

1 frozen waffle (not whole wheat), topped with butter or plain yogurt

1 cup decaf herbal tea

■ LUNCH

1 baked potato with sour cream

1 cup vegetables, such as broccoli, steamed or sautéed with 1 table-spoon of butter or olive oil

■ DINNER

1 bowl chicken soup with white rice—made with 2 cups of chicken broth, 4 ounces diced roasted chicken, 1 cup cooked rice, ½ cup of carrots

## DAY 4

■ BREAKFAST

4 ounces fruit juice (not grape)

1 plain bagel with butter

1 cup decaf tea

■ LUNCH

1 turkey sandwich on white bread with mayonnaise and mustard

■ DINNER

1 bowl of pasta (not whole wheat) with ⅓ cup tuna or 3 ounces of salmon tossed with olive oil and well-cooked vegetables

■ DAILY SNACKS

Graham or plain crackers

White bread or rolls

Pretzels

Plain or vanilla yogurt

After up to four days, proceed to Phase 2: The Diet for Mild to Moderate Back Pain.

## PHASE 2: DIET FOR MILD TO MODERATE BACK PAIN

This is the beginning of the healthiest time of your life! For the next three weeks, you will be eating the optimal diet designed to eliminate toxic build-up and bring your body back into balance, which will result in increased energy, better resistance to illness, greater mental ability, and reduced aches and pains. Your body will feel less stiff and more limber after just 21 days.

# Sample Meals

### DAY 1

■ BREAKFAST

1 egg plus 2 egg whites, scrambled in 1 teaspoon of olive oil

1 slice whole grain toast with ½ teaspoon butter

½ grapefruit

■ LUNCH

1 medium-size tossed salad (no croutons or cheese) topped with grilled chicken or tuna (no mayonnaise)

2 tablespoons oil and vinegar dressing

■ DINNER

1 bowl of whole grain pasta tossed with 1 tablespoon olive oil and crushed fresh garlic to taste

Grilled or steamed mixed vegetables with white beans

■ SNACK

½ cup mixed berries with 1 tablespoon crushed walnuts

## DAY 2

■ BREAKFAST

1 cup low-fat plain yogurt

¼ cantaloupe

1 slice whole grain toast with 1 teaspoon nut butter

■ LUNCH

1 slice whole grain bread topped with sliced turkey breast, lettuce, tomato, and 1 teaspoon mayonnaise

1 cup low-fat cottage cheese

■ DINNER

3 to 4 ounces lean steak, grilled or broiled

1 small side salad (vegetables only) with balsamic vinegar

½ baked sweet potato (can substitute white potato)

Steamed broccoli or mixed vegetables

■ SNACK

½ cup unsweetened applesauce mixed with ¼ cup whole grain cereal, sprinkled with cinnamon

## DAY 3

■ BREAKFAST

1 cup plain cooked oats (old-fashioned rolled or quick) with ½ cup diced apple and 1 tablespoon crushed walnuts, sprinkled with cinnamon

■ LUNCH

Mixed greens with assorted vegetables, topped with lean turkey, ham and natural cheese and drizzled with 2 tablespoons oil and vinegar dressing

1 very small whole grain roll or 1 slice whole grain bread

■ **DINNER**

1 broiled chicken breast, seasoned with lemon, garlic, onions, and parsley

Mixed vegetables (roasted with 1 tablespoon olive oil)

½ cup brown rice or quinoa

■ **SNACK**

½ cup pineapple (fresh or canned in own juice) with a dollop of low-fat plain yogurt, sprinkled with 1 teaspoon crushed walnuts

## DAY 4

■ **BREAKFAST**

1 whole grain English muffin topped with 1 poached egg, 1 slice Canadian bacon or lean turkey, and sliced tomato

Apple, sliced and sprinkled with cinnamon

■ **LUNCH**

Roasted vegetable sandwich made with ½ cup roasted mixed veggetables and 1 slice cheese, on 2 slices of whole grain bread spread with hummus

■ **DINNER**

6 ounces lean ground turkey or beef (at least 94% lean) mixed with unsweetened tomato sauce and vegetables (onions, peppers, and mushrooms)

1 bowl of whole wheat or brown rice pasta

■ **SNACK**

½ cup unsweetened granola

## DAY 5

■ **BREAKFAST**

Oatmeal with 2 tablespoons chopped walnuts and sliced pear, sprinkled with cinnamon

½ cup skim or unsweetened soy milk

■ LUNCH

Chef's salad made with mixed greens, turkey, ham, cheese, and raw vegetables, dressed with oil and vinegar

Whole wheat English muffin with hummus

■ DINNER

Roasted pork tenderloin

Baked sweet potato topped with cinnamon and a dollop of plain yogurt

Broccoli sautéed in garlic and olive oil

■ SNACK

Unsweetened applesauce, sprinkled with cinnamon

## DAY 6

■ BREAKFAST

1 whole grain bagel or 1 slice of whole grain bread

1 tablespoon almond butter

6 ounces plain nonfat yogurt with ½ cup mixed frozen organic berries, sprinkled with cinnamon

■ LUNCH

Cooked lentils mixed with quinoa, spinach, and crushed peanuts

Seasoned grilled tofu

1 bowl vegetable soup made with low-sodium stock (vegetable or chicken) and fresh or frozen vegetables

■ DINNER

1 poached chicken breast

Brown rice

Roasted root vegetables

## DAY 7

■ BREAKFAST

Oat bran flakes mixed with puffed wheat cereal

½ cup skim or soy milk

½ cup strawberries

2 tablespoons raw almonds

■ LUNCH

Avocado and black bean roll-up made with 1 oat bran tortilla spread with thin layer of nonfat yogurt, avocado, black beans, salsa, and brown rice

Add grilled chicken or tofu, if desired

■ DINNER

1 bowl vegetable soup (leftover from yesterday's lunch)

6 ounces grilled lamb chops

Spinach and garlic, stir-fried in 1 tablespoon olive oil

½ cup brown rice

## DAY 8

■ BREAKFAST

Whole wheat English muffin spread with cottage cheese and sprinkled with cinnamon

Sliced apple

1 egg, scrambled

■ LUNCH

Turkey chili

Whole grain roll

Small side salad with 2 tablespoons oil and vinegar dressing

■ **DINNER**

Grilled or broiled wild salmon brushed with 1 teaspoon olive oil

Quinoa tossed with diced apples and sunflower seeds in 1 tablespoon of walnut oil

Steamed or grilled asparagus sprinkled with Parmesan cheese

## DAY 9

■ **BREAKFAST**

Omelet made with 1 egg plus 2 egg whites with spinach, red peppers, and organic skim mozzarella cheese, cooked in 1 teaspoon canola oil

2 slices whole wheat toast with trans-fat free margarine or butter

■ **LUNCH**

Whole wheat pita pocket filled with chopped seasoned grilled chicken, roasted peppers, and mixed field greens and drizzled with 1 tablespoon of olive oil and balsamic vinegar

■ **DINNER**

Filet mignon

Wild rice

Roasted vegetables tossed with 1 tablespoon olive oil

## DAY 10

■ **BREAKFAST**

Yogurt parfait made with 6 ounces plain nonfat yogurt, chopped fruit, sunflower seeds, chopped walnuts, cinnamon, high-fiber dry cereal, a splash of soy milk, and a sprinkle of flaxseed

■ **LUNCH**

Grilled cheese sandwich made with 2 slices whole grain bread, 1 slice of Swiss cheese, 1 slice light Havarti cheese, sliced tomato, and baby spinach

1 cup roasted red pepper and tomato soup (or other vegetable or vegetable-bean soup)

■ DINNER

1 broiled chicken breast seasoned with lemon, garlic, and paprika topped with salsa and a dollop of plain yogurt

Grilled onions, peppers, zucchini, and mushrooms

½ cup brown rice

## Snack Ideas

- ► 6 ounces nonfat plain Greek yogurt with ½ cup blueberries and 1 tablespoon chopped walnuts

- ► 22 almonds

- ► 4 walnut halves and 4 dried apricot halves

- ► 1 cup cubed cantaloupe topped with ⅓ cup low-fat cottage cheese and cinnamon

- ► 3 cups popcorn tossed with 1 teaspoon olive oil and ¼ teaspoon chili powder

- ► 1 whole grain crisp bread cracker topped with ¼ avocado and 1 slice tomato

- ► 1 ounce cheddar cheese and ½ pear

- ► 1 whole grain crisp bread topped with 1 tablespoon almond butter and cinnamon

Follow similar meal plans for the next 11 days. Note after which meals you felt great and how your bowels responded. Reuse recipes or create similar ones based on foods that you enjoyed eating and also made you feel good, and eliminate those meals that left you gassy, bloated, or feeling too full. Listening to the signs of your own body will help you choose the remaining meals you make for the rest of Phase 2.

# PHASE 3: MAINTENANCE

After three weeks, you should be feeling a significant reduction in your back pain, as well as fewer digestive symptoms such as gas, bloating, diarrhea, constipation, and upset stomach. Your inflammation has been calmed, but you don't want to return to all your old ways—or you'll be back to where you started in just three weeks. It's important to maintain the basic framework of healthful input, so that you continue efficiently outputting and keep inflammation levels at a low. You'll probably find that when you waver and indulge in a little too much dessert or wine, your body will direct you back to your new healthy ways by speaking to you with a stiff back or a funny tummy. Stay in tune, and you'll naturally look for a balance of foods that make you feel great and can be eaten and enjoyed for the rest of your life!

## Basic Action

The maintenance period allows you to reintroduce some of the foods you were required to remove during the first three weeks. Ultimately, restriction doesn't do anyone any good. Just as you learned that too much of even the healthiest foods is not good for your body, neither is restriction. You shouldn't have sugary desserts or rich pasta dishes along with glasses of wine every day, but you also shouldn't forego foods that are especially appealing, especially on special occasions. Nor should you overdo any one food group, even vegetables. You must always seek balance. The No More Back Pain Diet has renewed your sense of well-being, and you want to focus on keeping that feeling.

During the Maintenance Phase, I highly recommend that you introduce foods one day at a time and keep a food journal and record the following:

- ▶ The amount of food you consumed

- ▶ The exact preparation of the food

- ▶ How you felt after each meal.

A food journal can speak volumes about your dietary habits and can help you see which particular foods or cooking methods create discomfort or pain.

## Duration

This is how you'll be eating from this day forward! By the time you've completed your three weeks of Phase 2, this approach will not seem overwhelming. You'll have learned what it feels like for your body to work optimally, and once you have reintroduced foods, you'll be aware of which ones you can occasionally enjoy and which are just too much for your system. You will most certainly be able to celebrate with a glass of wine and partake in birthday cake. Remember, balance and moderation is the key to maintenance, not restriction!

# THE ELIMINATION DIET

You know your back pain is due to digestive distress and you may have tried the No More Back Pain Diet. Perhaps you felt a little bit better but unfortunately, you didn't see a significant enough drop in your symptoms. That tells us something bigger is at play here—possibly a food allergy that needs to be eliminated entirely to help reset your system and keep it allergen-free going forward. An elimination diet is used to determine whether or not certain foods may be causing your symptoms or making them worse. You may suspect dairy, for instance, causes a problem for you, but you haven't given yourself the opportunity to remove it and reintroduce in a controlled way. The Elimination Diet is the way to get answers from your body about the causes of your digestive and back upset.

I have used elimination with many patients and have seen some miraculous results. For some people, the answer turned out to be the green drinks that they were sipping every morning. For others, it was their protein bars, or coffee, dairy or even beer. In its simplest form, the Elimination Diet removes things that you think may be causing your digestive upset, as well as things that you tend to be eating or drinking often on a consistent basis. What's important to remember when testing your body in this way is not to judge foods on the traditional "healthy" vs "un-healthy" model, but rather to judge them on how you specifically feel after you eat them. Broccoli is a much healthier food than a bagel; however, in this elimination diet, switching from a broccoli/kale drink for breakfast to a whole grain bagel could be the missing step to a back pain-free existence.  The elimination diet can simply be a diet hypothesis, based on clues from your body, leading to your food culprit, or it can be a removal of all the foods that you think could be potential allergens. Many of my patients have been resistant to this diet because they may have to give up their favorite foods or drinks. Telling my Canadian hockey player to stop drinking beer was not the easiest conversation! My response is always, "Let's try it for two weeks. If you don't feel better, that wasn't the answer. But if you do feel better, then you can figure out if you are able to enjoy it in moderation, if a different type doesn't trigger the same inflammatory response, or if you need to switch to something else entirely. The goal is just to get your back functioning better!"

There are four main steps to an elimination plan:

## STEP 1—Planning

Start by keeping a diet journal for a week, listing the foods you eat and jotting down the symptoms you have throughout the day. It is helpful to ask yourself a few questions:

- ▶ What foods do I eat most often?

- ▶ What foods do I crave?

- ▶ What foods do I eat to "feel better"?

- ▶ What foods would I have trouble giving up?

Often these foods seem to be the very ones that are most important to try not to eat. An occasional glass of wine might not cause back pain, but a glass or two every night might if you are sensitive to it, so it's important to be attentive to common allergens that are a part of your everyday lifestyle.

## STEP 2—Avoiding

The most common food proteins that can cause intolerance are cow's milk protein and gluten from wheat. Other foods that may be wreaking havoc in your gut are:

- ▶ Fatty meats like beef, pork, or veal. Leaner meats like chicken, turkey, lamb, and cold-water fish, such as salmon and trout, are usually more easily digested and can be eaten on the Elimination Diet, unless you know you are sensitive to them. While most

THE NO MORE BACK PAIN DIET

any fish is healthful, the major benefit of cold-water fish is that they are high in healthy Omega-3 fats. Choose organic/free-range sources where available.

▶ Alcohol and caffeine and all products that may contain these ingredients (including sodas, cold preparations, and herbal tinctures).

▶ Foods containing yeast or foods that promote yeast overgrowth, including processed foods, refined sugars, cheeses, commercially prepared condiments, peanuts, vinegar, and alcoholic beverages.

▶ Simple sugars such as candy, sweets, and processed foods.

For two weeks, you will eliminate the suspect food or foods, both whole or as ingredients in other things, without any exceptions. If you are using the diet to help resolve your Irritable Bowel Syndrome, consider eliminating all of the following foods for two weeks: dairy (lactose), wheat (gluten), high fructose corn syrup, sorbitol (chewing gum), eggs, nuts, shellfish, soybeans, beef, pork, and lamb, and reintroducing them one by one to detect the ones that are troublesome for you. The Elimination Diet for Irritable Bowel Syndrome can be found at the end of this chapter. If you don't have IBS and are doing the elimination diet to test for one or more food or food groups specifically, the following chart will help you identify which foods you are allowed and which ones to avoid within a particular allergen food group during the Avoidance Phase.

| FOOD GROUP | ALLOWED | AVOID |
|---|---|---|
| Meat, Fish, Poultry | Chicken, Turkey, Lamb, Cold Water Fishes such as Tuna and Salmon | Red meat, processed meats, smoked fish, eggs, and egg substitutes |
| Dairy | Rice, soy, and nut milks | Milk, cheese, ice cream, yogurt, frozen yogurt, butter, cream |
| Legumes | All legumes (beans, lentils) | None |
| Vegetables | All | Creamed or processed |
| Starches | Potatoes, rice, buckwheat, millet, quinoa | Products with gluten and corn (pastas, breads, chips) |

*(continued on next page)*

*(continued from previous page)*

| FOOD GROUP | ALLOWED | AVOID |
|---|---|---|
| Breads/Cereals | Any made from rice, quinoa, amaranth, buckwheat, teff, millet, soy or potato flour, arrowroot | All made from wheat, spelt, kamut, rye, barley |
| Soups | Clear, vegetable-based | Canned or creamed |
| Beverages | Fresh or unsweetened fruit/ vegetable juices, herbal teas, filtered/spring water | Dairy, coffee/tea, alcohol, citrus drinks, sodas |
| Fats/Oils | Cold/expeller pressed, unre-fined light-shielded canola, flax, olive refined oils, salad dressings, pumpkin, sesame, and walnut oils | Margarine, shortening, butter, and spreads |
| Nuts/Seeds | Almonds, cashews, pecans, flax, pumpkin, sesame, sunflower seeds, and butters from allowed nuts | Peanuts, pistachios, peanut butter |
| Sweeteners | Brown rice syrup, fruit sweeteners | Brown sugar, honey, fructose, molasses, corn syrup |

The elimination step takes a lot of discipline. In addition to utilizing the above chart, you must be particularly careful when eating out and you must also pay close attention to food labels. A number of foods can be disguised; when you look at food labels, beware of these things in the five major allergen categories:

| IF YOU ARE AVOIDING | ALSO AVOID |
|---|---|
| Dairy | Caramel candy, carob candies, casein and caseinates, custard, curds, lactalbumin, goat's milk, milk chocolate, nougat, protein hydrolysate, semisweet chocolate, yogurt, pudding, whey. Also beware of brown sugar flavoring, butter flavoring, caramel flavoring, coconut cream flavoring, "natural flavoring," Simplesse. |

| IF YOU ARE AVOIDING | ALSO AVOID |
|---|---|
| Peanuts | Egg rolls, "high-protein food," hydrolyzed plant protein, hydrolyzed vegetable protein, marzipan, nougat, candy, cheesecake crusts, chili, chocolates, and sauces. |
| Egg | Albumin, apovitellin, avidin, bernaise sauce, eggnog, egg whites, flavoprotein, globulin, hollandaise sauce, imitation egg products, livetin, lysozyme, mayonnaise, meringue, ovalbumin, ovogyco-protin, ovomucin, ovomucoid, ovomuxoid, Simplesse. |
| Soy | Chi-fan, ketjap, metiauza, miso, natto, soy flour, soy protein concentrates, soy protein shakes, soy sauce, soybean hydroly-sates, soby sprouts, sufu, tao-cho, tao-si, taotjo, tempeh, textured soy protein, textured vegetable protein, tofu, whey-soy drink. Also beware of hydrolyzed plant protein, hydrolyzed soy protein, hydrolyzed vegetable protein, natural flavoring, vegetable broth, vegetable gum, vegetable starch. |
| Wheat | Atta, bal ahar, bread flour, bulgar, cake flour, cereal extract, couscous, cracked wheat, durum flour, farina, gluten, graham flour, high-gluten flour, high-protein flour, kamut flour, laubina, leche alim, malted cereals, minchin, multi-grain products, puffed wheat, red wheat flakes, rolled wheat, semolina, shredded wheat, soft wheat flour, spelt, superamine, triticale, vital gluten, vitalia acaroni, wheat protein powder, wheat starch, wheat tempeh, white flour, whole-wheat berries. also beware of gelatinized starch, hy-drolyzed vegetable protein, modified food starch, starch, vegetable gum, vegetable starch. |

Many people notice that in the first week, especially in the first few days, their symptoms will become worse before they start to improve. If your symptoms become severe or increase for more than a day or two, consult your doctor.

## STEP 3—Challenging

If your symptoms have not improved in two weeks, stop the diet and talk with your doctor about whether or not to try it again with a different combination of foods. However, if your symptoms do improve, start "challenging" your body with the eliminated foods, one food group at a time. As you do this, keep a written record of your symptoms.

To challenge your body, re-add the eliminated food, starting with just a small amount in the morning. If you don't notice any symptoms, eat two larger portions in the afternoon and evening. After a day of eating the new food, remove it, and wait for two days to see if you notice the symptoms re-arise.

If a food doesn't cause symptoms during a challenge, it is unlikely to be a problem food and can be added back into your diet at the end of the Elimination Test. Don't add the food back right away until you have tested all the other foods on your potential-allergen list. Keeping your diet bland and allergen-free while you search for your trouble-maker will ensure that small flair-ups don't arise.

If a food causes you to have an immediate allergic reaction, such as throat swelling, a severe rash, or other severe allergy symptoms, seek medical care immediately and avoid food challenges unless you are directly supervised by a physician.

Some people have problems with more than one food, and you will need to first cleanse your body of all those foods and reintroduce them in phases. Here is an example of an Elimination Diet Calendar that includes the removal procedure for diary, wheat and caffeine.

| DAY NUMBER | STEP |
| --- | --- |
| 1 | Begin Elimination Diet of all foods that seem to be potential allergens |
| 2-7 | Symptoms may worsen for a day or two |
| 8-14 | Symptoms should go away if the right foods have been removed |
| 15 | Re-introduce food #1, dairy (do not yet re-introduce wheat or caffeine) for just one day. |

| DAY NUMBER | STEP |
|---|---|
| 16-17 | Stop dairy intake and watch for symptoms. Even if your old symptoms do not arise and you feel dairy may not have been the culprit after all, you will not add it back into your meal plan until the entire elimination diet is over. |
| 18 | Re-introduce food #2, wheat. |
| 19-20 | Stop wheat intake and watch for symptoms. |
| 21 | Re-introduce food #3, caffeine. |

Be sure that you are getting adequate nutrition during the elimination diet. For example, if you give up dairy, you must supplement your calcium from other sources like leafy green vegetables. You also want to be sure to drink at least two quarts of water a day to keep your colon flushed out and to allow your bowels to properly excrete.

## STEP 4—Creating a New, Long-Term Diet

Based on your results, you'll have a list of foods that do not agree with your body. Whether this is a short list or a longer list, it's important that you find foods that provide similar nutrients to the foods you'll be permanently eliminating. For dairy, alternatives may include calcium and vitamin D-fortified nut or seed milks and yogurts, and high calcium foods like tofu processed with calcium, broccoli, leafy greens, sesame seeds, and canned fish with bones. For a peanut intolerance, opt instead for other nuts and seeds, like almonds, hazelnuts, cashews, sunflower seeds, or hemp seeds. If you're unable to eat eggs, make sure that your breakfasts still include a source of protein, such as yogurt or tofu (if you're allowed soy/dairy) or a nut/seed butter like almond butter or hemp seed butter. If soy was a symptom trigger for you, then you should be getting lean protein in your diet through foods like beans, lentils, fish, chicken, and grass-fed beef. And finally, if you can no longer eat wheat, opt for a wheat-free grain like buckwheat, quinoa, barley, teff, amaranth, or millet. It is recommended that you speak with a doctor or registered dietitian to analyze your symptoms and create a meal plan that ensures you are still getting all the nutrients you need now that you have removed one or more foods or food groups from your daily intake.

# Elimination Diet for IBS Sufferers

This diet is for those with IBS, who should eliminate ALL foods known to be allergens and begin with a very basic, plain diet. This allows the stomach to heal and will help you identify all the food sensitivities that you may have.

■ BREAKFASTS

### HOT CEREAL WITH BANANA SLICES

2 cups cooked cream of rice cereal prepared with water and
    2 tablespoons of trans-fat-free margarine (Promise spread is good!)

Top with sliced banana

### COLD CEREAL WITH RICE MILK

2½ cups puffed rice cereal with 1½ cups plain or vanilla low fat rice milk

### BREAKFAST POTATO WITH CINNAMON APPLESAUCE

1 medium baked potato (no skin) with 1½ cups unsweetened applesauce
    mixed with cinnamon

■ LUNCHES

### GRILLED CHICKEN WITH RICE

6 ounces grilled chicken breast with 1½ cups cooked white rice mixed
    with 1 tablespoon of trans-fat-free margarine

### TURKEY BURGER WITH BAKED POTATO

6 ounces plain turkey burger with 1 medium baked potato topped with
    2 teaspoons of soft tub margarine (no potato skin)

### TURKEY AND AVOCADO ON RICE CAKES

6 ounces sliced turkey breast (or grilled chicken) divided over 3 plain rice
    cakes, each topped with 1 slice avocado
Eat with ½ cup unsweetened applesauce

■ DINNERS

## TURKEY WITH MASHED POTATO

6 ounces turkey breast with 1 medium baked potato mashed with
1 tablespoon of margarine and 1 cup white rice

## GRILLED FISH WITH RICE

8 ounces grilled salmon, sole, trout or tilapia with 1 teaspoon olive oil and
1 cup white rice
Chicken with Baked Potato
5 ounces chicken with baked potato topped with 1 tablespoon margarine
(no skin)

■ SNACKS

1 cup unsweetened applesauce
1 small banana
3-5 plain rice crackers
2 plain rice cakes
1 ounce baked potato chips (make sure they do not include Olestra).
½ baked potato with 1 teaspoon margarine (no skin)


After following this meal plan for three weeks, you will actually realize
that your back pain was a gift. It was the way your body communicated,
telling you how it wanted you to eat, and allowing you to not only resolve
your back problems, but also makeover your digestive system as well.
When your cravings kick in, remember this: changing what you eat is
the easiest and could be the most profound thing that you can do for
your back. Ultimately, improper nutrition for everyone's unique digestive system is the unidentified cause for millions of back pain sufferers. A
relief from pain isn't the only benefit. You'll also have more energy and a
better functioning digestive system. Before you undertake any aggressive
back pain treatments, make sure that you have eliminated your current
diet as the cause!

# FODMAPS DIET:
# AN ALTERNATIVE ELIMINATION PLAN

Another elimination diet to help with the symptoms of Irritable Bowel Syndrome is called FODMAPs, a plan low in fermentable oligo-, di-, and monosccharides and polyls (FODMAPs), which limits foods that contain:

- ► **Lactose**—found in milk, ice cream, yogurt, and cheese
- ► **Fructose**—found in fruits such as apples, pears, peaches, mangos, and berries
- ► **Fructans**—found in wheat, onions, garlic, asparagus, cauliflower, mushrooms
- ► **Galactans**—found in beans and lentils
- ► **Sugar Alcohols (polyols)**—found in honey, agave, high-fructose corn syrup, sorbitol, mannitol, Splenda, and other sweeteners

These compounds in food can be poorly absorbed, leading to increased water and gas in the GI tract, and thus distention, bloating, and discomfort. To assess your tolerance for these compounds, eliminate foods high in FODMAPs for six to eight weeks. Then, reintroduce one food every four days with a two-week break in between bothersome foods. Be careful to eat just small portions of each food group when adding back into your diet. Ideal test amounts are:

- ► **Lactose:** ½-1 cup milk
- ► **Fructose:** ½ mango or 1-2 teaspoons honey
- ► **Fructans:** 2 slices wheat bread, 1 garlic clove or 1 cup pasta
- ► **Galactans:** ½ cup lentils or chickpeas
- ► **Sugar Alcohols:** Sorbitol, 2-4 dried apricots; Mannitol, ½ cup mushrooms

This will help you identify the threshold at which you are able to consume FODMAP-containing foods without causing your GI symptoms to reappear.

# 10

# IT MIGHT BE THE WAY YOU MIX

## Principles of Food Combining and Digestive Health

Most of you are accustomed to thinking about the quality of food in terms of its individual components (such as good carbs versus bad carbs), or the quality of diet in terms of its overall composition (such as low carb, low fat, or low calorie foods). But the *combination* of different foods can also affect how you feel and how much you weigh.

Do you have any of these symptoms?

- ▶ Recurrent bowel problems, especially gas or bloating

- ▶ Chronic stomach upset

- ▶ Indigestion/routine use of digestive aids

- ▶ Feeling uncomfortably full long after you've eaten

- ▶ Unexplained weight gain

If you've completed three weeks of the No More Back Pain Diet, but are still feeling symptomatic, learning about the principles of food combining could be your solution! It was for me!

I always felt bloated, full and nauseated after meals. For a long time, I lived with this sensation and assumed it was just normal. But after about a decade of feeling weighed down after eating, rather than re-energized, I visited Dr. Goodheart, the same doctor who helped identify the digestive source of my father's back pain. Dr. Goodheart was one of the first people to use food combination to ease digestive ailments and told me that my food choices were not the problem (they were healthy!), but the way I was combining these foods was causing my discomfort.

Here's the easy medicine behind food combination: different foods require different digestive environments. Eating foods with similar digestive needs improves the efficiency of digestion and leaves you feeling rejuvenated and alive after consuming them. Conversely, eating foods that require different digestive environments (as I was doing) leads to inefficient digestion and a bloated, stuffed, tired feeling.

It took a while for me to get used to a new way of eating, but the feeling I now have after I eat has changed my life. I created The Food Combination Diet to make the principles of food combination easy to incorporate into everyday life, and I recommended it to friends and patients who were also feeling that post-meal discomfort (which should only be reserved for Thanksgiving Day!). The diet relieved their symptoms within three weeks too, and unwanted weight seemed to come off without much effort.

Here are my simple principles of food combining:

## PRINCIPLE 1: EFFICIENT EATING, EFFICIENT DIGESTION
### Food combinations that favor efficient digestion

Although our bodies are designed to digest mixed meals (meals that contain a combination of starch, protein, and fat), many people respond to meals in a more efficient way when their bodies can focus on one type of food at a time. Different types of foods need different digestive environments to be digested efficiently, which maximizes the amounts of nutrients we can take from food. Even people who can digest mixed meals with few problems find that eating foods in the appropriate combination increases their energy, reduces gas and bloating, and helps them maintain a healthy weight.

There are two major reasons why the improper combination of foods can lead to impaired digestion:

1. **Opposing digestive environments:** Proteins and starches need very diverse environments to be digested efficiently. Foods that are made mostly of protein (such as meat and eggs) begin digestion in the stomach, which is very acidic. Starchy foods like bread and pasta require an alkaline, or basic, environment and need to be digested before and after they are in the stomach. When we eat foods that require two different digestive environments at the same time, the process becomes inefficient, leaving undigested food in the stomach. This results in bloating or gas. Eating a meal comprised of all foods that are digested in the same way allows your body to focus on creating the ideal environment for thorough, efficient processing.

2. **Poor digestive timing:** Food gets mixed together upon entering the stomach and is then released into the small intestine, the next section of the digestive tract. The rate that your stomach releases this mixture into the small intestine is highly dependent on the composition of the food you just ate. If there is a lot of fat in this mixture when it enters the small intestine, your body sends signals to your stomach to release the rest more slowly. This delay in stomach emptying is useful for protein, which needs more time in the acidic stomach to digest. However, it does not work so well for fruit, which quickly breaks down into gas-producing substances if forced to remain in the stomach for too long because it has been mixed with other foods. For this reason, fruit should always be eaten on its own!

Now that you are familiar with the basic science behind food combining, you're ready to apply this knowledge as you learn how to combine specific foods to maximize your digestive potential.

## PRINCIPLE 2: IT'S NOT THE FIVE FOOD GROUPS ANYMORE

The Food Combination Diet uses seven categories of food based on digestive properties in order to optimize the way your body can process what you consume, help you lose weight, and promote overall wellness.

## CATEGORY 1: Starches

This group consists of:

- ▶ Breads (white, wheat, multigrain, English muffins)
- ▶ Grains (rice—both brown and white, barley, oats, millet, quinoa, bulgur, spelt, rye, buckwheat, amaranth)
- ▶ Starchy vegetables (corn, white potatoes, sweet potatoes, yams, winter squash—butternut and acorn, peas, water chestnuts, parsnips, and pumpkin)

## CATEGORY 2: Proteins

- ▶ Meats (fish, chicken, pork, lean beef)
- ▶ Eggs
- ▶ Beans (kidney, white, cannelloni, chickpea or garbanzo, black, pinto, lentils, red, navy)
- ▶ Soy (tofu, tempeh, edamame)
- ▶ Cheese

## CATEGORY 3: Non-Starchy Vegetables

- ▶ Bell peppers, onions, asparagus, cabbage, eggplant, endive, artichokes, arugula, broccoli, broccoli rabe, brussels sprouts, green beans, spinach, watercress, zucchini, celery, carrots, shallots, mushrooms, rhubarb, cauliflower

## CATEGORY 4: Milk and yogurt

- ▶ Milk (skim, 2%, acidophilus, fortified, soy milk)
- ▶ Yogurt (nonfat plain, low-fat plain, nonfat Greek, 2% Greek)

## CATEGORY 5: Nuts, seeds, and nut and seed butters

- ► Nuts (peanuts, almonds, walnuts, pine nuts, pistachios, macadamia, pecans, brazil nuts, hazelnuts, cashews, soy nuts)

- ► Seeds (sunflower or pumpkin)

- ► Nut and seed butters (peanut, almond, sunflower, soy nut, or cashew)

## CATEGORY 6: Fruit

## CATEGORY 7: Fats and Oils

- ► Vegetable oils (olive oil, canola oil, sesame oil, coconut oil, grape seed oil)

- ► Solids (butter, margarine, Crisco)

- ► Condiments (mayonnaise, salad dressings, sesame seeds)

Now you know the seven food groups. The user-friendly Combining Guide on on page 167-168 tells you which foods you can combine and will make it easy to create digestively effective meals. Here's how to use the chart:

### Meal categories (1-4)

Creating simple meals by picking the right combinations from groups 1 through 4 allows you to eat a diet that includes all of the nutrients you need, while achieving optimal digestive timing and food combinations. These meal combinations will keep you satisfied and energetic until your next snack or meal.

### Snack categories (5-7)

Due to the specific timing and combination of foods in this diet, snacks are important and will ensure that you get the nutrients you need. You should include fruit in your diet because it's high in fiber, vitamin, minerals, and can improve digestion. You should strive for at least two servings of fruit a day, but eat it alone, thirty minutes before other foods (remember, fruit moves rapidly through your digestive tract!). Fruit is great to eat as a digestive primer before meals!

# PRINCIPLE 3: START SMALL AND PHASE IN NEW COMBINATIONS

The Food Combination Diet has been broken down into three phases in order to accommodate differing digestive capabilities. Everyone should begin with the most digestively gentle phase, Phase 1. Not everyone will progress to Phase 3; in fact, some people will find the most digestive comfort by remaining in Phase 1. Most people will find ideal digestive balance in Phase 2, but there are many who find they fall somewhere in between phases. For example, someone in Phase 1 might tolerate one or two combinations from Phase 2.

Phase 1 adheres to the strictest principles of food combining in order to rejuvenate and restore balance to your digestive system. Although everyone should begin with Phase 1, your digestive system will act as a guide and let you know when you are ready to move on to the next phase. I recommend you stay on Phase 1 for at least two symptom-free weeks (i.e., no gas, bloating, uncomfortable fullness after eating, etc.). This allows your body and mind to adjust to a new way of eating. When you are ready to move into Phase 2, you can begin combining some starches and proteins and trying small portions of fruit with other easily-digestible foods. It is best to add one new combination a week to make it easier to identify which food combinations are problematic to you. While you will be finding a dramatic reduction in back and digestive pain by week 3, stay in Phase 2, symptom free, for at least six weeks before adding in any Phase 3 combinations.

## PHASE 1: Digestive rejuvenation period (2+ weeks)

- ▸ Balances the digestive system
- ▸ Creates an ideal internal environment for efficient digestion of each food category
- ▸ Minimizes gas, bloating, and toxic buildup
- ▸ Brings the body closer to optimal metabolism and nutrient utilization

## PHASE 2: Maintenance and strengthening (6+ weeks)

► Builds and maintains a strong digestive system

► Allows a wider variety of food combinations

## PHASE 3: Strong digestion

► Provides the widest variety of food combinations

► Introduces these combinations slowly and one at a time

Even in Phase 3, I try to avoid the "Meat and Potatoes" plates which cause me the most upset. Your Phase 3, or your Lifetime Phase, will also likely include meals that are predominantly protein or predominantly starch, but each stomach is unique so be attentive as you test your combinations. What is nice about this diet is you might not have to give up some of your favorite foods at all—you just have to know how and when to eat them. So go and enjoy your spaghetti and meatballs, just don't eat them together!

| COMBINING GUIDE | | | | |
|---|---|---|---|---|
| | FOOD CATEGORY | COMBINE WITH | | |
| | | Phase 1 | Phase 2 | Phase 3 |
| 1 | Starches: breads grains, cereals, starchy veggies (potatoes, sweet potatoes) | Non-starchy veggies, fats | Fruit, Rice with beans | |
| 2 | Proteins: meats, eggs, beans, tofu, tempeh, cheese | Non-starchy veggies, fats | Beans with rice | |

*(continued on next page)*

*(continued from previous page)*

| COMBINING GUIDE | | | | |
|---|---|---|---|---|
| | **FOOD CATEGORY** | **COMBINE WITH** | | |
| | | Phase 1 | Phase 2 | Phase 3 |
| 3 | Non-starchy veggies | Starches, starchy veggies, meats, nuts, eggs, fats, oils and grains | Fruit | Milk, yogurt |
| 4 | Milk, Yogurt | Fats | Fruit | Non-starchy veggies |
| 5 | Nuts and nut butters | | Non-starchy veggies, fruit | |
| 6 | Fruit | | Milk, yogurt, non-starchy veggies | |
| 7 | Fats and Oils | Non-starchy veggies, starches, starchy veggies | | |

## PRINCIPLE 4: TIMING IS EVERYTHING

Proper timing of meals and snacks allows you to get the most nutrients out of the foods you eat and achieve and maintain optimal digestion. You want to allow just enough time between meals and snacks for your food to completely leave your stomach—but not so much time that you get too hungry. In order to ensure that your last meal or snack has been efficiently digested, wait two hours between meals and snacks and thirty minutes between a fruit snack and a meal. Timing meals this way prevents the mindless between-meal munching that leads to weight gain. It also keeps your energy level stable throughout the day.

Here's the ideal timing for daily food consumption. The mid-morning and mid-afternoon snacks are included to prevent over-eating at meals and to help you listen to your own fullness cues.

| | |
|---|---|
| 8 a.m. | Breakfast |
| 10 a.m. | Snack |
| 12 p.m. | Fruit |
| 1 p.m. | Lunch |
| 3 p.m. | Snack |
| 6 p.m. | Dinner |
| 8 p.m. | Snack (optional) |

## PRINCIPLE 5: DON'T FORGET QUALITY AND VARIETY

The quality and wholesomeness of the foods you eat is important. You want to choose whole foods over processed ones. For example, by making a stir fry over a whole grain like quinoa, bulgur, brown rice, or whole wheat pasta rather than over white rice or white pasta, you'll be getting more fiber, protein, vitamins B and E, minerals, copper, magnesium, zinc, and selenium. Whole grains, along with fruits and vegetables, also contain plant substances called phytochemicals. These compounds, which give fruits and veggies their vibrant colors, are often lost during processing and offer a wide variety of health benefits, from disease prevention to pain relief. Phytochemicals and other bio-active compounds in whole foods cannot be replaced once processing has removed them.

Eating a variety of foods not only increases the number of different phytochemicals and other nutrients in your diet, it also makes eating more exciting and pleasurable. Making a list of combinations you like, along with ones you want to try, can be a great way to prevent combination monotony and ensure variety. Add to your list often, using each addition as a reminder to vary your combinations and experiment!

Aside from having less fiber and nutrients, processed foods are often loaded with salt, unhealthy fats, and chemicals that can contribute to toxic build-up in the body. Too much sodium can leave you bloated, your skin looking lackluster, and can be dangerous if you already tend to have high blood pressure. Trans-fat, a type of fat used in processed foods to increase shelf life, can increase your risk of heart disease. And some people are particularly sensitive to chemical additives which can cause headaches and loss of energy.

The Food Combination Diet limits processed foods in your diet; however, you also need to make good choices. Cooking and preparing your meals with fresh, whole foods may require more work, but once your body realizes how good it feels, you won't want to go back to your old eating habits. The recipes that I've provided will help you get creative while you adhere to the four principles of food combination! Your stomach—and your back!—will thank you!

## FOOD COMBINATION DIET

Even after you know the new meal categories and the principles of Food Combination, it can take a while to figure out meals and snacks that are both interesting and adhere to the plan. It did for me! But now I can share my diverse Food Combination meal plan, created with help of Willow Jarosh from C&J Nutrition, with guidance for Phases 1 and 2. Easy recipes follow the plan!

## PHASE 1

### DAY 1

■ BREAKFAST

1 Oatmeal Flax Muffin (see recipe)

■ SNACK

Four 6-inch celery sticks

2 tablespoons peanut butter

■ FRUIT

1 medium piece of fruit (or ½ cup non-mixed fruit)

■ **LUNCH**

Mixed vegetable stir fry with chicken—4 ounces chicken, 2 cups mixed vegetables

■ **SNACK**

1 ounce whole grain crackers

2 tablespoons hummus

1 medium piece of fruit (or ½ cup non-mixed fruit)

■ **DINNER**

1 serving Baked Halibut (see recipe)

1 ½ cups vegetables

■ **EVENING SNACK**

6 ounces plain nonfat or low-fat Greek yogurt with cinnamon (optional)

## DAY 2

■ **BREAKFAST**

Broccoli and cheese omelet (2 eggs or equivalent egg substitute, ⅓ cup chopped, cooked broccoli, 1 ounce shredded cheddar cheese)

■ **SNACK**

1 granola bar (cinnamon, flax, oats, and honey)

■ **FRUIT**

1 medium piece of fruit (or ½ cup non-mixed fruit)

■ **LUNCH**

Roasted vegetable and hummus wrap (one 8-inch whole-wheat tortilla, ¾ cup roasted vegetables, ½ cup mixed greens, 2 tablespoons hummus)

■ **SNACK**

⅓ cup Neutralization Trail Mix (see recipe)

■ **DINNER**

1 serving Greek Stuffed Chicken (see recipe)

■ EVENING SNACK

8 ounces steamed almond or soy milk (heated in saucepan to steaming point) with 1 teaspoon vanilla and a dash of cinnamon

## DAY 3

■ BREAKFAST

1 serving Tofu Scramble (see recipe)

■ SNACK

1 cup plain cereal

■ FRUIT

1 medium piece of fruit (or ½ cup non-mixed fruit)

■ LUNCH

One 6-9 piece vegetable sushi roll

1 cup miso soup

1 seaweed salad

■ SNACK

⅓ cup Neutralization Trail Mix

■ FRUIT

1 medium piece of fruit (or ½ cup non-mixed fruit)

■ DINNER

1 serving Broiled Salmon with Rosemary and Lemon

5 spears roasted asparagus sprinkled with 1 tablespoon Parmesan cheese

■ EVENING SNACK

1 serving Rice Pudding (see recipe)

## DAY 4

■ BREAKFAST

1½ cups hot cereal, cooked (made with water), cinnamon (optional)

■ SNACK

Four 6-inch celery sticks

2 tablespoons peanut butter

■ FRUIT

1 medium piece of fruit (or ½ cup non-mixed fruit)

■ LUNCH

Grilled chicken salad (4 ounces grilled chicken, 2 cups mixed greens, 2 tablespoons oil and vinegar dressing)

■ SNACK

1 Oatmeal Flax Muffin (see recipe)

■ DINNER

1 serving Tempeh Napoleon (see recipe)

■ EVENING SNACK

6 ounces Greek style yogurt

## DAY 5

■ BREAKFAST

1 serving Greek Egg Scramble (see recipe)

■ SNACK

⅓ cup Neutralization Trail Mix

■ FRUIT

1 medium piece of fruit (or ½ cup non-mixed fruit)

■ LUNCH

1 serving Tempeh Napoleon (see recipe)

■ SNACK

1 serving Rice Pudding (see recipe)

■ FRUIT

½ cup melon or other fruit

■ DINNER

1 serving beef or pork tenderloin (see recipe)

1 cup cooked vegetables

■ EVENING SNACK

8 ounces steamed milk with cocoa powder and vanilla


## DAY 6

■ BREAKFAST

1 serving Eggs Florentine (see recipe)

■ SNACK

1 Oatmeal Flax Muffin (see recipe)

■ FRUIT

½ cup mixed melon salad

■ LUNCH

Beef tenderloin and baby spinach salad (use beef tenderloin from previous night's diner)—3 ounces sliced beef tenderloin, ½ cup mixed chopped green and red peppers, ¼ cup red onion, ¼ cup reduced fat shredded cheese)

■ SNACK

Granola bar (cinnamon, flax, oats, and honey)

■ DINNER

1 serving Sprouted Grain Pasta (see recipe)

■ EVENING SNACK

1 medium apple sliced and sprinkled with cinnamon

## DAY 7

■ BREAKFAST

1 Oatmeal Flax Muffin (see recipe)

■ SNACK

6 ounces plain yogurt

■ FRUIT

1 medium piece of fruit (or ½ cup non-mixed fruit)

■ LUNCH

4 ounces grilled chicken

2 cups grilled vegetables

■ SNACK

1 ounces string cheese

1 cup baby carrots or carrot sticks

■ FRUIT

½ cup melon

■ DINNER

1 serving Grilled Vegetable Pizza (see recipe)

Side salad with:

- ► 1½ cups raw salad with veggies
- ► 1 tablespoon of oil and vinegar

■ EVENING SNACK

½ cup pineapple chunks

½ cup sliced strawberries (4 whole berries)

# PHASE 2

### DAY 1

■ BREAKFAST

Berry Parfait

6 ounces plain nonfat yogurt

1 cup mixed berries (can be frozen)

1 tablespoon ground flaxseed

■ SNACK

1 Granola Bar

■ FRUIT

1 medium piece of fruit (or ½ cup non-mixed fruit)

■ LUNCH

1 serving Mexi-rice (see recipe)

■ SNACK

1 ounce baked tortilla chips

¼ cup guacamole (without tomatoes)

■ FRUIT (if needed)

1 medium piece of fruit (or ½ cup non-mixed fruit)

■ DINNER

4 ounces chicken stir fried with 1 cup broccoli

■ EVENING SNACK

1 Vegan Carrot Muffin (see recipe)

1 cup herbal tea

## DAY 2

- **BREAKFAST**

  2 frozen whole-grain waffles topped with ½ cup frozen blueberries (thawed) (those in phase 3 can use bananas)

- **SNACK**

  ¼ cup mixed nuts

- **FRUIT**

  ½ cup chopped cantaloupe or other melon

- **LUNCH**

  4 ounces broiled fish with 1 cup cooked vegetables

- **SNACK**

  1 mini bag or ½ regular bag of 94% fat-free microwave popcorn

- **FRUIT**

  1 medium piece of fruit (or ½ cup non-mixed fruit)

- **DINNER**

  Baked bell pepper stuffed with Mexi-rice

- **EVENING SNACK**

  ½ cup cottage cheese

## DAY 3

- **BREAKFAST**

  1 serving Citrus Smoothie (see recipe)

- **SNACK**

  1 Vegan Carrot Muffin (see recipe) (Carrot raisin muffin for Phase 3)

- **LUNCH**

  Salad with grilled vegetables

> ▸ 1 cup leafy greens
> ▸ 1 cup grilled vegetables
> ▸ ¼ cup shaved cheese

■ AFTERNOON SNACK

1 ounce pita chips

¼ cup hummus

■ FRUIT

1 medium piece of fruit (or ½ cup non-mixed fruit)

■ DINNER

4 ounces pork tenderloin

1 cup steamed carrots

■ EVENING SNACK

1 ounce whole grain crackers

## DAY 4

■ BREAKFAST

1½ cups hot cereal, cooked (prepared with water) and ⅓ cup mixed frozen berries

■ SNACK

1 cup raw veggies

1 ounce string cheese

■ LUNCH

4 ounces grilled, broiled, or baked chicken with 1 cup cooked veggies

■ SNACK

1 cup ready to eat whole grain cereal (no sugar added)

■ FRUIT

¼ cup dried apricots

■ **DINNER**

1 serving Whole Wheat Penne with Broccoli and Mushrooms

■ **EVENING SNACK**

6 ounces all natural fruited low/non-fat yogurt

## DAY 5

■ **BREAKFAST**

1 serving Vegetable Omelet (see recipe)

■ **SNACK**

1 Vegan Carrot Muffin (see recipe)

■ **FRUIT**

1 medium piece of fruit (or ½ cup non-mixed fruit)

■ **LUNCH**

1½ cups penne pasta dish from night before

■ **SNACK**

1 ounce string cheese

■ **FRUIT**

¼ cup dried cranberries

■ **DINNER**

1 serving Broiled Salmon (see recipe from Phase 1)

6 spears roasted asparagus

■ **EVENING SNACK**

6 ounces all natural low/non-fat fruited yogurt

## DAY 6

■ **BREAKFAST**

Two 4-inch Pancakes with Apple Cinnamon Topping (see recipe)

■ SNACK

½ cup cottage cheese

■ LUNCH

1 serving Mediterranean Pasta Salad (see recipe)

■ FRUIT

1 cup sliced watermelon

■ DINNER

1 serving shrimp sauté

■ EVENING SNACK

1 mini bag or ½ regular bag 94% fat free microwave popcorn

## DAY 7

■ BREAKFAST

Scrambled eggs—1 egg plus 1 white (or equivalent egg substitute) scrambled with ⅓ cup onions and mushrooms and 2 tablespoons shredded cheese

■ SNACK

6 ounces low or non-fat fruited yogurt

■ LUNCH

Bagel Sandwich—whole grain bagel spread with 2 tablespoons hummus and topped with 1 grilled portabella mushroom cap, ¼ cup sprouts, and 2 large slices roasted pepper

■ SNACK

1 Vegan Carrot Muffin (see recipe)

■ FRUIT

1 medium piece of fruit (or ½ cup non-mixed fruit)

■ DINNER

1 serving Greek Stuffed Chicken (see recipe)

■ EVENING SNACK

1 slice whole grain toast with 1 teaspoon light butter or margarine

Tea

## DAY 8

■ BREAKFAST

1½ cup hot cereal, cooked (prepared with water), with ⅓ cup sliced peaches

■ SNACK

1 ounce part skim string cheese

1 cup raw vegetables

■ LUNCH

Roasted vegetable salad—¾ cup roasted vegetables over 2 cups green salad tossed with 1 tablespoon vinaigrette

Whole Grain Roll

■ SNACK

1 ounce baked pita chips

■ FRUIT

½ cup sliced melon

■ DINNER

4 ounces grilled halibut with ½ cup roasted green and yellow zucchini

■ EVENING SNACK

8 ounces steamed almond or soy milk (heated in saucepan to steaming point, with 1 teaspoon vanilla and dash cinnamon)

## DAY 9

■ BREAKFAST

Yogurt berry parfait—8 ounces plain low or non-fat yogurt layered with ½ cup berries (fresh or frozen)

■ SNACK

⅓ cup Neutralization Trail Mix

■ FRUIT

1 medium piece of fruit (or ½ cup non-mixed fruit)

■ LUNCH

4 ounces lean beef with 1½ cups veggies

■ SNACK

1 Vegan Carrot Muffin (see recipe)

■ DINNER

Lentils with rice—add ¾ cup cooked brown rice to 8 ounces canned vegetarian lentil soup

■ SNACK

½ cup pineapple chunks

## DAY 10

■ BREAKFAST

1 serving vegetable frittata

■ SNACK

1 medium apple (sliced), dipped in 4 ounces low/nonfat Greek or regular yogurt

■ LUNCH

Grilled tuna salad—4 ounces tuna (can use pre-seasoned vacuum pack tuna steaks) over 1½ cups mixed greens and ½ cup chopped mixed vegetables (bell pepper, onion, celery, mushrooms)

■ SNACK

1 ounce wholegrain crackers with 2 tablespoons hummus

■ FRUIT

½ cup sliced melon

■ DINNER

1 serving Sprouted Grain Pasta Ribbons (see recipe)

■ EVENING SNACK

1 Vegan Carrot Muffin (see recipe)

## DAY 11

■ BREAKFAST

1½ cups hot cereal, cooked with water, with ⅓ cup chopped apple and cinnamon

■ SNACK

6-8 ounces low/nonfat fruited yogurt

■ LUNCH

One 6-9 piece vegetable sushi roll

8 ounces miso soup

Green side salad with ginger dressing

■ SNACK

½ cup cottage cheese

■ FRUIT

½ cup cantaloupe with ¼ cup berries

■ DINNER

4 ounces roasted chicken with 4 ounces cooked brussels sprouts

■ SNACK

1 ounce pita chips

## DAY 12

■ BREAKFAST

Two 4-inch whole-grain frozen waffles with ½ cup sliced peaches

■ **SNACK**

1 serving lemon dill yogurt (see recipe)

1 cup raw vegetables

■ **LUNCH**

Grilled chicken salad—4 ounces grilled chicken on 2 cups mixed greens with 2 tablespoons vinaigrette

■ **SNACK**

¼ cup mixed nuts

■ **FRUIT**

1 medium piece of fruit (or ½ cup non-mixed fruit)

■ **DINNER**

1 serving Tofu Asian Vegetable Stir-fry (see recipe)

■ **EVENING SNACKS**

1 medium apple, baked with cinnamon and 2 tablespoons raisins

### DAY 13

■ **BREAKFAST**

1 serving Greek Egg Scramble (see recipe)

■ **SNACK**

1 ounce part skim milk string cheese

■ **LUNCH**

Portabella mushroom wrap—4 inch portabella mushroom grilled and sliced, ½ cup greens, ¼ cup sautéed onions in a 10-inch whole wheat tortilla

■ **FRUIT**

½ cup sliced melon

■ **SNACK**

1 granola bar

■ DINNER

1 serving Sautéed Scallops (see recipe)

6 spears steamed asparagus

■ EVENING SNACK

1 serving Poached Pear with Vanilla and Cinnamon (see recipe)

## DAY 14

■ BREAKFAST

Yogurt Berry Parfait—8 ounces low/nonfat yogurt layered with ½ cup berries (fresh or frozen)

■ SNACK

1 carrot muffin

■ LUNCH

Smoked turkey roll ups over green salad

3 slices turkey spread with 1 tsp hummus, topped with ½ slice light (or thinly sliced regular) Swiss cheese and rolled up. Place on top of 2 cups mixed greens tossed with 2 tablespoons vinaigrette dressing.

■ SNACK

¼ cup mixed nuts

■ FRUIT

1 medium piece of fruit (or ½ cup non-mixed fruit)

■ DINNER

1 serving vegetable won tons (see recipe)

■ EVENING SNACK

½ bag or 1 single-serving bag microwave popcorn

# RECIPES

Okay, so now you know the phases and the foods you can eat during each one. Here are the simple recipes so that you can follow the plan and whip up proper plates at home!

## PHASE 1

■ BREAKFAST ■

### OATMEAL FLAX MUFFINS

¼ cup milled flaxseed

⅔ cup rolled oats

1 cup natural white flour

2 teaspoons baking powder

½ teaspoon baking soda

½ teaspoon salt

3 tablespoons vegetable oil

½ cup rice milk

¼ cup molasses

2 teaspoons cinnamon

1 teaspoon vanilla

DIRECTIONS

Preheat oven to 400 degrees. Blend dry ingredients together in a large mixing bowl. In separate bowl, combine oil, rice milk, molasses, and vanilla. Add dry ingredients to wet mixture and mix until fully blended. Batter will be thick. Line medium sized muffin tin with liners. Spoon about ⅓ cup of batter into tins and bake for 18-20 minutes or until top springs back when touched. Remove from pan and cool on wire rack. **MAKES 6 MUFFINS**.

### GREEK EGG SCRAMBLE

2 whole eggs*

2 tablespoons water

2 tablespoons olives

1 tablespoon crumbled feta cheese

1 tablespoon finely chopped scallions

¼ cup chopped mushrooms

Pinch of salt and pepper to taste

### DIRECTIONS

Beat eggs and water in small bowl with whisk. Stir in salt, pepper, scallions, and olives; set aside. Place medium non-stick skillet or sauté pan over medium-high heat. Cover bottom of pan with cooking spray and add mushrooms. Sauté mushrooms for about 30 seconds until lightly browned. Pour egg mixture into pan. Reduce heat to medium. Slowly scramble the mixture. When eggs are mostly set but still slightly wet add crumbled feta cheese. Continue to cook until eggs are set but moist. **SERVES 1.**

*1 egg = 2 egg whites = ¼ cup egg substitute

## EGGS FLORENTINE

1 or 2 whole eggs*

1 cup fresh or ½ cup frozen spinach prepared according to package directions

2 teaspoons shredded parmesan cheese

Salt and pepper to taste

### DIRECTIONS

Grease 1 quart saucepan with cooking oil. Half fill the pan with water. Bring water to boiling; reduce heat to simmering (bubbles should begin to break the surface). Break one egg into a measuring cup. Slide egg into simmering water, carefully holding the lip of the measuring cup as close to the water as possible. Simmer eggs uncovered for three to five minutes until whites are set and yolks begin to thicken but are not hard. Remove eggs with a slotted spoon. Season with salt and black pepper. Serve poached egg over steamed or sautéed spinach. Top with shredded parmesan cheese. **SERVES 1.**

*1 egg = 2 egg whites = ¼ cup egg substitute

## TOFU SCRAMBLE

⅕ block firm or extra firm tofu, cubed

¼ cup chopped sweet onion

¼ cup chopped red bell pepper (fresh or frozen)

Salt and pepper to taste

Dash of cumin and chili powder

Canola oil cooking spray

### DIRECTIONS

Heat medium non-stick skillet over medium-high. Cover bottom of pan with cooking spray. Add onions and sauté for 1 minute. Add remaining ingredients and spices. Stir frequently until tofu is golden brown for four to five minutes. **SERVES 1.**

■ LUNCH ■

## ROASTED VEGETABLES

1 small zucchini, cut into ⅓ inch slices

1 small eggplant, cut into ⅓ inch slices

1 red onion, peeled, and cut into ¼ inch slices

1 red pepper, cored, and cut into 1 inch strips

2 portobello mushroom caps, cut into 1 inch slices

3 large carrots, cut in half lengthwise, and then into 3 or 4 inch strips

2 teaspoons dried oregano

1 teaspoon chopped fresh thyme (or ½ teaspoon dried)

2 tablespoons olive oil

½ teaspoon pepper

Pinch of salt

### DIRECTIONS

Preheat oven to 400 degrees F. Brush bottom of large baking pan with olive oil. Arrange all vegetables (choose as many types as you like) on baking pan. Brush top of vegetables with olive oil and sprinkle herbs, salt, and pepper evenly. Bake on middle oven rack for about 20-25 minutes, or until vegetables are tender and slightly browned. Turn vegetables halfway through baking. You can add fresh rosemary or any other herb to change the recipe to your liking. **SERVES 4.**

## TEMPEH NAPOLEON

8 ounces tempeh

2 tablespoons olive oil

1⅓ cup roasted vegetables

Salt and pepper to taste

4 tablespoons Parmesan cheese

### DIRECTIONS

Preheat oven to 400 degrees. Slice the tempeh in half, widthwise. Then cut each half, lengthwise, into eight slices. In a nonstick skillet over medium-high heat, heat the olive oil. When the oil is hot, add the tempeh and cook until browned on both sides for three to four minutes per side. Remove from heat and sprinkle lightly with salt and pepper. On a baking sheet, place four slices of tempeh side by side. Place ⅓ cup of roasted vegetables on top of the tempeh and sprinkle with 1 tablespoon Parmesan cheese. Place four more pieces of tempeh on top of the vegetables. Place ⅓ cup more vegetables and 1 tablespoon of cheese on top of the second layer of tempeh. Repeat this procedure to make a second Napoleon, using the remaining eight pieces of tempeh, vegetables, and cheese. Bake in the oven for ten minutes. **SERVES 2.**

▪ DINNER ▪

## SPROUTED GRAIN PASTA

2 cups sprouted grain pasta ribbons, cooked (available at most natural food stores, Trader Joe's, Whole Foods, etc.)

1 cup cremini mushrooms, chopped

2 cups fresh baby spinach

½ cup vegetable broth

2 cloves garlic

Fresh ground pepper

2 tablespoons olive oil, separated

### DIRECTIONS

Cook sprouted grain pasta according to package directions, drain and toss with 1 tablespoon of olive oil. Heat oil in large skillet on medium high heat. Sauté garlic for 30 seconds. Add spinach and stir until wilted for about one minute. Add olives and mushrooms and sauté for an additional minute. Stir in broth and simmer for an additional five minutes. Stir in pasta and mix thoroughly. Place pasta dish in bowl and top with freshly ground pepper. **SERVES 2.**

## BAKED HALIBUT

1 6-ounce Halibut steak

⅛ cup vegetable broth

2 teaspoons lemon juice

1 garlic clove, pressed

1 tablespoon capers

2 teaspoons chopped fresh parsley (optional)

1 teaspoon fresh tarragon, chopped (optional)

1 teaspoon chopped fresh chives (optional)

Salt and pepper to taste

DIRECTIONS

Preheat the oven to 450 degrees. Place halibut steak in small baking dish. Combine broth, lemon juice, garlic, capers, and herbs and pour over fish. Bake for 15 minutes or until fish flakes with a fork. Pour remaining pan juices over fish and enjoy. **SERVES 1.**

## GREEK STUFFED CHICKEN

One 4 ounce chicken breast

1 teaspoon lemon juice

1 teaspoon dried oregano

Dash salt and pepper

1 teaspoon olive oil

## STUFFING

2 tablespoons crumbled feta

2 tablespoons chopped Kalamata olives

2 tablespoons chopped onion

¼ cup chopped spinach

DIRECTIONS

Start by combining all stuffing ingredients in a large bowl. With knife parallel to cutting board, make a deep three-inch long cut in the center of the chicken breast to form a pocket. Stuff the center of the chicken breast with the stuffing mixture. Combine lemon juice, oregano, olive oil, salt and pepper and pour over chicken breast. Bake at 350 for 45 minutes. SERVES 1.

## CARMELIZED ONION AND ROASTED VEGETABLE PIZZA

1 12-inch whole-wheat pizza crust

1 medium red bell pepper, cut lengthwise into eighths

1 medium zucchini, cut into ¼ inch slices

1 medium onion, thinly sliced (about 1 cup)

½ small eggplant cut into ¼ inch slices

1 tablespoon fresh basil leaves

2 tablespoons olive oil

Pinch of salt

Freshly ground pepper

DIRECTIONS

Preheat oven to 425 degrees. Lightly spray baking sheet with cooking spray. Line sheet with all vegetables except onion; brush lightly with 1 teaspoon olive oil and sprinkle with salt and pepper. Bake vegetables on middle rack for about 20 to 25 minutes or until vegetables are tender.

While vegetables are roasting, heat 1 tablespoon olive oil in skillet over medium heat. Reduce heat to low; add onions, sauté until golden brown, about 15 minutes. Brush pizza shell with 1 teaspoon olive oil. Spread onion mixture evenly over bottom of pizza. Top with roasted vegetables. Bake an additional eight to ten minutes. Sprinkle fresh basil over top of pizza if desired. SERVES 4.

## BEEF TENDERLOIN STEAKS WITH HERBED MUSHROOM SAUCE

½ pound beef tenderloin, cut into two 4-ounce steaks

2 teaspoons Dijon style mustard

1½ cups mixed wild mushrooms (can use cremini, shitake, portabella, or button)

¼ cup dry red wine or sherry

1½ teaspoons Worcestershire sauce

1½ teaspoons olive oil

1 teaspoon fresh thyme (or ¼ teaspoon dried)

½ teaspoon fresh rosemary (⅛ teaspoon dried rosemary)

### DIRECTIONS

Trim any visible fat from the tenderloin steaks. Spread mustard evenly over both sides of the steaks. Heat 2 teaspoons oil in large skillet over medium-high heat. Add steaks and reduce heat to medium. Cook to desired doneness (seven to nine minutes for medium-rare to medium). Transfer to serving platter but keep meat warm.

Add remaining 1 teaspoon oil to skillet. Add mushrooms; cook and stir for four minutes. Stir in wine, Worcestershire sauce, rosemary and thyme. Simmer, uncovered for about three minutes. Spoon over steaks and serve. **SERVES 2.**

## BROILED DILL SALMON

1 4-6 ounce fresh or frozen salmon filet

2 teaspoons finely chopped dill (or ½ teaspoon dried)

⅛ teaspoon sea salt

Pinch of pepper

2 lemon wedges

### DIRECTIONS

Preheat oven to 350 degrees. Coat baking sheet with cooking spray; lightly coat fish with cooking spray. Sprinkle dill, salt and pepper over fish. Squeeze juice of one lemon wedge over fish. Bake for 10 minutes or until fish flakes with a fork. **SERVES 1.**

■ SNACKS ■

## NEUTRALIZATION TRAIL MIX

    1 cup raw or dry roasted unsalted almonds

    1 cup dried cranberries

Mix together. **MAKES 8 SERVINGS.**


## RICE PUDDING

    4 cups water

    ¾ cup short grain white rice

    4 cups rice milk

    1 teaspoon ground cinnamon

    1 teaspoon vanilla

    1 teaspoon freshly grated lemon or orange peel

### DIRECTIONS

Bring water to a boil in a saucepan. Once boiling, add the rice and simmer for five minutes. Drain rice and return to the pan with the rice milk, cinnamon, vanilla, and lemon peel. Bring mixture to a boil. Reduce the heat and gently simmer for 40-50 minutes, stirring often. The mixture will become thick and creamy. Remove from heat and allow to sit for five minutes before serving. Sprinkle with additional cinnamon, if desired. Can be served warm or chilled. **SERVES 6.**

# PHASE 2

When you are ready to progress to Phase 2, you can incorporate more foods and add different combinations. Here are some of my favorite recipes, included in your Phase 2 meal plan, for you to try!

■ BREAKFAST ■

## VEGAN CARROT MUFFINS

¾ cup all-purpose flour

½ cup wheat germ

½ cup whole wheat flour

½ teaspoon baking powder

¼ teaspoon baking soda

¼ teaspoon ground nutmeg

¼ teaspoon ground cloves

1 teaspoon cinnamon

1 cup finely grated carrot

¼ cup unsweetened applesauce

8 ounces unsweetened apple juice

### DIRECTIONS

Preheat oven to 400 degrees. In a large mixing bowl combine the flours, spices, baking soda, baking powder, and grated carrot. In a separate bowl, combine the applesauce and juice. Pour the liquid ingredients into the dry ingredients and stir until just combined. Place muffin liners in a muffin tin and spoon ⅓ cup of batter into each cup. Bake in the oven for 15-20 minutes, or until the tops begin to brown. Remove from the pan and cool thoroughly on a wire rack. **MAKES 6 MUFFINS.**

## CITRUS SMOOTHIE

8 ounces plain low/nonfat yogurt

4 ounces all natural orange juice

3 large, whole strawberries, chopped

1 kiwi, peeled and chopped

Ice cubes

### DIRECTIONS

Place all ingredients in a blender and blend until smooth. Serves 1.

## PANCAKES WITH APPLE-CINNAMON TOPPING

1 medium apple, cored and sliced

½ teaspoon cinnamon

½ cup apple juice

½ teaspoon orange or lemon zest

½ teaspoon vanilla extract

### DIRECTIONS

Place apple slices, juice, zest, and cinnamon into a saucepan. Bring to a boil, then quickly turn down the heat and simmer until apples are tender. If more liquid is needed, add some water. Once apples are tender, add vanilla. Prepare pancakes using your favorite recipe or whole grain pancake mix. Spoon apple mixture over pancakes. **SERVES 2.**

## VEGETABLE FRITTATA

¼ cup diced onion

⅓ cup bell pepper and/or zucchini

⅛ teaspoon salt

Pinch coarsely ground black pepper

2 teaspoons finely chopped fresh basil

1 egg plus 1 egg white

1 tablespoon water

1 tablespoon feta cheese, crumbled

Nonstick vegetable cooking spray

### DIRECTIONS

Add onion to a small nonstick skillet coated with cooking spray. Cook over medium-high heat until golden. Add peppers, zucchini, salt, and pepper. Cook, stirring frequently, until tender. Remove from heat; stir in the basil. In a medium bowl, beat the egg and water. Pour the egg mixture over the vegetables in the skillet and cook over medium-high heat until the egg becomes firm. Flip the frittata onto a plate and then back into the pan and cook until the underside is golden brown. Sprinkle with feta cheese. **SERVES 1.**

## FIESTA RICE

½ cup canned black beans, drained

1 cup brown rice, cooked

¼ cup chopped green peppers

¼ cup chopped onions

1 tablespoon olive oil

⅛ teaspoon cumin

⅛ teaspoon paprika

salt and pepper to taste

DIRECTIONS

Prepare rice according to directions. Pour olive oil into a nonstick skillet. Add the chopped onions and cook over medium heat until slightly tender for about a minute. Add the green peppers to the onions and cook for an additional two to three minutes. Turn heat down to low and add black beans, spices, and salt and pepper (if desired) to the vegetable mixture. Stirring frequently, cook until heated through. Once the mixture is heated, add the rice to the skillet and mix. Remove from heat. **SERVES 1.**

## MEDITERRANEAN PASTA SALAD

½ cup roasted peppers

4 marinated artichoke hearts (oil packed—reserve 2 tablespoons liquid), drained and coarsely chopped

¼ cup olives, coarsely chopped

Pinch of pepper

2 cups cooked whole wheat penne or other pasta

DIRECTIONS

Cook pasta according to instructions on package. In a large bowl, add reserved liquid from the artichokes to the pasta and mix to coat. Add the peppers, artichoke hearts, olives and peppers to the mixture and toss. **SERVES 2.**

■ DINNER ■

## WHOLE WHEAT PENNE WITH BROCCOLI AND MUSHROOMS

1 cup cooked broccoli (from fresh to frozen)

1 cup mushrooms, thickly sliced

2 cups cooked whole wheat penne

1½ tablespoons plus 2 teaspoons olive oil

¼ teaspoon chopped garlic

¼ teaspoon ground dried oregano

Pinch of salt and pepper

DIRECTIONS

Combine olive oil, salt, pepper, oregano, and garlic in the bottom of a large bowl and set aside. Add 2 teaspoons olive oil to a nonstick pan. Add the mushrooms and cook over medium-high heat until tender. Add the broccoli to the mushrooms and cook for an additional minute. Remove vegetables from the heat. Add the cooked, drained penne and the vegetables to the olive oil and herb mixture and toss to coat. **SERVES 2.**

## VEGETABLE WON TONS

¼ cup finely chopped cabbage

¼ cup grated carrot

¼ cup finely chopped mushrooms

1 green onion, chopped

½ clove garlic, chopped

Pinch red pepper flakes

1 tablespoon soy sauce

2 teaspoons sesame oil (can use canola oil)

½ cup vegetable broth or water

12 small won ton wrappers

Nonstick cooking spray

DIRECTIONS

Combine all ingredients, except won ton wrappers, in a large bowl. Place 1 tablespoon of the filling mixture in the center of a won ton wrapper. Lightly brush the edges of the wrapper with water and bring the four corners together in the center. Pinch the edges together to form a small packet that seals in the filling. Coat the bottom of a nonstick pan with cooking spray and cook the won tons over medium-high heat until the bottoms are golden brown. Pour ½ cup vegetable broth or water into the pan, cover and steam for about two minutes or until much of the liquid has evaporated and thickened. **SERVES 2**.

## SHRIMP SAUTÉ

4 ounces medium-sized shrimp
½ teaspoon chopped garlic
⅓ cup snow peas
⅓ cup bok choy
⅓ cup baby corn
2 teaspoons canola oil
1 teaspoons sesame oil (optional)
Pinch of salt and pepper
Pinch red pepper flakes

### DIRECTIONS

Heat canola and sesame oil in a nonstick skillet over medium-high heat. Add garlic vegetables, salt, pepper, and pepper flakes and cook until tender for about two to three minutes. Add the shrimp and cook until it turns pink. **SERVES 1**.

## TOFU ASIAN VEGETABLE STIR-FRY

⅕ block tofu
⅓ cup snow peas
⅓ cup bok choy
⅓ cup baby corn
¼ cup chopped onion
2 teaspoons canola oil
1 teaspoon sesame oil (optional)
Pinch salt
Pinch pepper
Pinch red pepper flakes

DIRECTIONS

Heat canola and sesame oil in a nonstick skillet over medium-high heat. Add onion, salt and pepper flakes and cook until tender (about 2 minutes). Add the tofu and cook until it begins to brown. Add the remaining vegetables and cook just until the bok choy wilts. **SERVES 1.**

## SAUTEED SCALLOPS

4 ounces scallops

⅓ cup white wine

1 teaspoon olive oil

1 teaspoon butter

1 tablespoon chopped fresh basil

Salt and pepper to taste

DIRECTIONS

Melt the butter and oil together over medium heat in a small skillet. When the butter and oil are hot, add scallops. Cook until browned (about two minutes) and then turn over and cook the second side until just browned. Add the white wine and simmer until the alcohol has evaporated (about two minutes). Remove from heat and sprinkle with basil.

## ROASTED ACORN SQUASH STUFFED WITH QUINOA, RAISINS, APRICOTS, APPLES, AND SPICES

1 medium-sized acorn squash

1 cup cooked quinoa

2 tablespoons golden raisins

2 tablespoons chopped dried apricots

½ cup chopped apples

⅛ teaspoon dried thyme

Salt and pepper to taste

Nonstick cooking spray

DIRECTIONS

Preheat oven to 400 degrees. Wash and dry the acorn squash. Slice a thick piece off both ends of the squash. Cut the squash in half lengthwise and scoop out the seeds with a spoon. Place the two halves, cut side down, in a baking dish sprayed with nonstick cooking spray. Bake for 45 minutes. While the squash is baking, combine quinoa, fruit, and seasonings in a bowl. Place half the quinoa mixture in each of the squash halves. Place the halves back into the oven for an additional 30 minutes. **SERVES 2.**

■ SNACKS ■

## POACHED PEARS WITH VANILLA AND CINNAMON

    1 teaspoon ground cinnamon

    ¼ teaspoon ground cloves

    ¼ teaspoon ground allspice

    1 cup dry white wine

    1 cup all natural apple juice (use 2 cups if you want to omit the
        wine)

    2 pears, cored

DIRECTIONS

Place wine and juice in a saucepan over medium heat. Add spices and bring to a boil, then turn heat to low. Add the pears and simmer for 10 minutes. Turn off heat and allow pears to sit in liquid for an additional 20 minutes. Serve each pear over Greek yogurt, with 1/4 cup of the cooking liquid. **SERVES 2.**

## LEMON-DILL YOGURT DIP

    8 ounces plain low/nonfat yogurt

    1 teaspoon dried dill

    ¼ teaspoon pepper

    1 teaspoon dried onion flakes

    1 tablespoon lemon juice

DIRECTIONS

Combine all ingredients and refrigerate in sealed container. Makes 2 servings.

# 11

# HONING IN ON YOUR HORMONES

## A SINETT STORY

Sometimes I hesitate to share my patients' stories because they can sound a bit off the wall and can create more skepticism about my work. However, since I'm introducing you to my theory of balance in the body and the idea that the entire body is connected, these stories really are essential in showing how the problem often isn't where it seems to be. I want to share one very personal story. Please realize fertility issues are not always this simple, but I promise every part of this account is true. Here's our story and its miraculous result:

•   •   •

My WIFE AND *I had been trying, unsuccessfully, to get pregnant for approximately eight months, and we were extremely frustrated because her menstrual cycle was so irregular, occurring about once every three months. She saw numerous gynecologists and took multiple prescription medications but saw no change. As time passed and our treatment options dwindled, our emotional stress spiked, not to mention the financial stress of spending hundreds of dollars a month on ovulation predictor kits, medications, and pregnancy tests! We finally turned to my father for help with our very private problem.*

*When my father examined my wife, he saw that her hormonal system was completely out of balance. He determined that the pituitary gland was not sending the proper messages to the rest of the hormonal organs. The pituitary gland is the conductor of the orchestra, he said, while the rest of the organs are the individual instruments. My dad's feeling was that no one was leading the orchestra. Something (or someone) needed to tell the conductor to raise the baton and get the instruments playing together.*

*My father started my wife's treatment by recommending an herbal and vitamin complex called Ovex, to support female androgen production and ovarian health and function. He then stimulated bones in my wife's head that impact the pituitary gland and treated numerous acupuncture points and specific drainage points that relate to the hormonal and digestive systems. Lastly, my father changed my wife's diet, taking away all of the simple sugars and simple carbohydrates in her diet. Within a week, my wife got her period and her cycle has been regular ever since. We got pregnant the next month and now have two beautiful children.*

*My father heard many similar stories, the results of which are simply too predictable to be described as coincidence. The simple act of achieving balance structurally, digestively, emotionally, and even hormonally, does wondrous and miraculous things to the body. It is what I strive to achieve each day by paying attention to the bigger picture in each and every one of my patients.*

If you answered yes to these questions, your back pain could be hormonally induced:

- ▶ Did you just begin your menstrual period or have you recently started menopause?
- ▶ Has your hormonal system undergone any recent changes (menopause, change in birth control, missed menstrual period, pregnancy, etc.)?

While men are susceptible to hormonal imbalance, women suffer from the majority of hormonal back pain. This shouldn't come as a surprise to most women who know that some level of back pain usually comes from PMS and the onset of menstruation.

A Swedish study even showed that women on birth control pills or hormone replacement therapy (HRT) are more likely to suffer from back pain, and as a result, European doctors have stopped prescribing the birth control pill if a woman is suffering from back pain to allow time for her hormones to even out.

Pregnancy is also a huge cause of back pain but it isn't just the extra weight that leaves the pregnant woman groaning. As many as half of all women experience back pain in the first trimester, before much weight has been gained at all! Hormones released during pregnancy allow the ligaments in the pelvic area to soften and the joints to become looser in preparation for giving birth, which directly affects the mother's back. Your Ob/gyn or internist may also be able to help you focus on your chemical imbalance and identify the right way to treat it.

Nutrition and vitamin imbalance can also throw off your hormones, resulting in back pain. While it's best to visit a nutritionist to identify where you are over- or under-producing hormones, general nutrition recommendations for getting hormones back into balance include:

1. Choose the least refined versions of carbohydrates (whole grains instead of bread, a bowl of steel cut oats instead of cereal; corn, peas, or winter squash in a soup instead of pasta).
2. Balance your carbs with protein at each meal. So if you want a baked potato, include a piece of chicken, fish, or beef with it.
3. Opt for healthful fats with each meal, such as nuts, seeds, nut butters, cold-pressed oils, avocado, and olives.
4. Limit your sugar intake, preferably to one small dessert a day at most! Reduce caffeine and alcohol as well. Anything that raises cortisol levels in the body can elevate the hormonal response. Thankfully the converse is true. I have patients who avoid alcohol for the two weeks prior to their menstrual cycle to help keep their hormones in check.

Acupuncture has also been helpful to rebalance the body's chi. Find a practitioner who is versed in both traditional and holistic approaches in hormonal balances.

If hormones are to blame for your back pain, visiting your gynecologist, obstetrician, endocrinologist, or internist can help. Any one of these doctors should be able to find out whether you have a chemical imbalance and the right way to treat it. Sometimes a trip to the nutritionist who can prescribe vitamins to balance your body and initiate proper function is all it takes!

# 12

# WHO TO SEE FOR DIGESTIVE ISSUES

**D**igestive issues are often resolved by changing what you put in your refrigerator and then, what you put in your mouth. But sometimes there are diseases such as Crohn's, IBS, or severe allergies that need attention. If you have back pain stemming from digestive issues, here is a list of doctors you should see or treatments to seek, starting with the least invasive.

## LEVEL 1: Self-help

If the Back Pain Inflammatory Index showed that your back pain is caused by a digestive imbalance, the first step is to look at what you are eating. Simply changing your unhealthy eating habits to healthy ones can make all the difference in the world. Remember, what is healthy for you is unique, and formulating your own plan based on the diet that is right for you will ensure both gastrointestinal and back pain relief in just three weeks. However, if you don't completely make the dietary changes, you may not give the body time to completely heal—so be consistent with the diet. A half-hearted effort means you'll probably conclude that your back pain wasn't nutritionally based. If you do the three week plan properly and still feel you are facing digestive upset, deeper allergies or stomach problems may be at work, and you should proceed to a Level 2 practitioner.

## LEVEL 2: See a nutritionist

While you may think that you have the knowledge or you can just assess yourself, most of you should see a nutritionist. A certified nutritionist has in-depth knowledge and training not just about foods and diets but on vitamins as well. A vitamin or mineral deficiency could be the cause of your back pain. Nutritionists can help guide you on specifically what foods to eat and what not to eat, as well as teach you how to analyze labels and even show you how to look at a menu and pick the proper foods when you're dining out. This can be tricky to do on your own, especially if you are someone who eats out frequently. You may have been making missteps in your Level 1 diet that you were unaware you were doing!

## LEVEL 3: Internist or gastroenterologist

If you have finished Levels 1 and 2 and have not gotten results, it is time to see your internist and/or a gastroenterologist. A specialist can examine you to make sure that there aren't any underlying issues or problems. These level 3 providers are great diagnosticians and can also prescribe the necessary medications to not only help with your digestive function but with your back pain as well. Unfortunately, the majority of these providers haven't received much training in diet and nutrition so make sure that you have completed Levels 1 and 2 first.

# THE THREE-WEEK TAKE-AWAY

## Three Easy Tips to Help You Target Your Digestive Solution

The suggestions in this chapter are designed to help you make small changes that can make a big difference in how you feel.

## 1. Kickstart your day!

Drink a large glass of cold water first thing in the morning. This should stimulate your digestive process and jump start your body's ability to eliminate your waste products. Remember, your back will only function as well as how your bowels function!

## 2. Listen to your body!

Your body speaks to you after eating. Rather than listening to what you know about healthy foods, listen to your body. How you feel and how you excrete is the best possible information on how your digestive system is working and how optimal your diet is for you.

## 3. Mix it up!

Too much of a good thing applies even to health food! Variety is a vital part in a good functioning digestive system. Make sure that you have at least three different breakfasts, lunches, and dinners in your rotation.

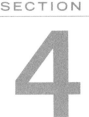
# Emotional Diagnosis and Solution

# 13

# THE FIRST STEP TO AN EMOTIONAL SOLUTION IS CREATING POSITIVE MENTAL CHANGES

Almost every day patients come to my office complaining of back or neck pain that I eventually diagnose as being caused by emotional or stress issues. If you scored 4 or more points in the Emotional Section of the Back Pain Inflammatory Index, your back pain is stemming, at least in part, from an emotional cause.

The best explanation that I've heard of what it means to be stressed comes from one of my patients who told me, "People who are stressed are no longer able to live in the moment. They are too worried about what has just happened and what's coming next to be able to live in—or enjoy— the present." Life stressors—and our often negative reactions to them in the form of anger, distress, or fear—are major triggers of both acute and chronic back and neck pain. The stress-induced muscle tightening that occurs during both waking and sleeping can result in debilitating physiological pain of the neck, shoulders, and back. Nervous stomach, headache, broken-out skin, and jaw pain are also very real physical problems, all of which have an emotional base.

I often hear doctors say that a patient's problems are all in his or her mind. This is true—but not how the doctors mean it. The mind and body are so interconnected that they actually make up one undivided network. Most people recognize that when something upsetting happens, it is normal to feel tense, sad or irritable. But when you experience a psychological imbalance, often you also develop a physiological imbalance or pain, such as a headache, cold, stomachache, or backache. These symptoms usually manifest several days after the difficult event, so you don't always make the connection.

• • •

*I FIRST VISITED the Midtown Integrative Health & Wellness office to seek help for a pain that I was experiencing in my lower back and down my left leg. The pain was bothering me particularly at night when I was lying down and sometimes even stopped me from sleeping. I didn't know what was causing it and thought a chiropractor could help. A friend told me about Dr. Sinett, and soon after I began seeing him, the pain in the lower back went away. Dr. Todd gave me back adjustments and I used the Backbridge™ in the office and at home. Even if the back pain came back occasionally, I would lie on the Backbridge™ or see Dr. Todd for an adjustment, and I would immediately feel better.*

*I continued to visit the office as I was finding his therapy very effective to release other tensions in my body. I was also training for the New York City marathon, and if I was very sore from a long run, Dr. Todd would adjust my legs and the pain would go away.*

*Seeing the great benefits on my body, we then started focusing more and more on my emotions. Dr. Todd uses a method, the NET technique, that was new to me, but I think it is the most effective way of freeing a patient from emotional tensions. He was able to help me identify what was bothering me by asking questions and testing the strength on my shoulder muscles. In my case, the problem area was always "love." I had gone through a difficult time in my marriage, which eventually led to separation and divorce, and I was going through the ups and down of dating. I found it difficult to reconcile the various steps of meeting a new guy and then choosing the right course of action in the craziness of a big city like New York. But the amazing thing about this method is that it lets your body tell you if your decisions and actions are congruent with your thoughts. At the same time, it allows you to go deeper into your emotions and understand what has led you to make certain choices that probably were not always beneficial for you. The process of healing the emotions took a bit longer than healing the back pain, but it was not any less successful. Over the years I learned to identify the patterns that were good for me and eventually found someone who loves and respects me and whom I love and respect. In finding love, I have also found more balance in my emotional health!*

*Sabrina Muheim*

When a patient is hit with back pain and the doctor can't find a structural cause, it often turns out that the pain is both a symptom and an expression of some distress in the person's life. Most people don't want to believe this explanation because they view it as a weakness or a flaw in their personality. We are programmed to think that we are supposed to be able to handle stress and that we should be tough enough to withstand sickness or pain from something emotional.

But the body is programmed to respond to emotional stress. When we are stressed, several things happen:

▸ Heart rate and blood pressure soar, increasing the flow of blood to the brain to improve decision making.

▸ Blood sugar rises to furnish more fuel for energy as the result of the breakdown of glycogen, fat, and protein stores.

▸ The blood is shunted away from the gut (and digestion stops so as not to use up energy that is needed elsewhere) and directed to the large muscles of the arms and legs in order to provide more strength in combat or greater speed in getting away from a scene of potential peril.

▸ Blood clotting occurs more quickly to prevent blood loss from lacerations or internal hemorrhage.

These and many other automatic responses occur, even though the nature of stress for modern humans is no longer confrontation with a saber-toothed tiger, but rather getting stuck in traffic or dealing with a family or work situation. Still, our bodies maintain that same fight-or-flight response, which, over time, can lead to chronic fatigue, digestive upset, headaches, and back pain.

Today, most people confront a steady barrage of medium-level stressors. This constant level of tension depletes our adrenal glands, and the body's constant call for adrenaline wears us out and leaves us ill-prepared to react to the next stressor we encounter. It also affects the body's ability to function in unison, which is why you might feel like your head is spinning from all that is going on. Internally, the systems of your body are spinning. Your muscles are only contracting and not relaxing, and your cerebrospinal fluid is flowing too fast, irritating the vagus nerve which controls our abdominal organs. This irritation causes all sorts of stress reactions, from brain freeze to an upset stomach.

## The Causes of Stress Reactions

Understanding the various types of stress can help you determine where your own stress comes from. This is the first step to resolving your emotionally induced back pain.

# INTERNAL PRESSURES AND EMOTIONAL CONFLICT

Emotional conflict and the pressures we place on ourselves frequently cause enough stress to manifest in back pain. Anytime we dread or don't want to do something, we can cause a physical reaction in our body. It isn't surprising that the greatest number of heart attacks occur on Monday mornings. People physically respond to the thought of the weekend being over and the start of the workweek.

I have many examples of patients who have suffered very real pain caused by internal and emotional conflict. I will share the stories of two of them.

Ken, a healthy, active 26-year-old, who had been under my care for a few years for some mild structural pain, was an ideal patient, coming in once a month for a chiropractic adjustment to make sure he stayed healthy. One day, Ken called and said he could barely get out of bed due to severe back pain. He blamed me and wanted to fire me. We talked on the phone long enough for me to encourage him to come into the office one more time so I could see what had happened. As I examined him, I could see he was truly suffering, but I couldn't find a structural explanation. I talked about how stress causes muscle tightness and ultimately terrible pain. Was he stressed about anything in particular? Ken had an "aha" moment. He said he was getting married in two weeks and had been having second thoughts. I encouraged him to do what he had to do to resolve his feelings—and his pain.

Ken said his back pain was the best thing that ever happened to him. He called off his wedding and hasn't had any back pain since.

A similar phenomenon occurred with a patient who came in to the office bent over with lower back pain so severe she had trouble getting on the examination table. While I was taking her case history, she mentioned that her father had died the previous summer and that summer had always been their time together. We determined that as spring was turning warmer, the change in seasons was triggering a negative anniversary stress response. I find this often happens with patients who are approaching the anniversary of a big break-up or death. Our minds take note of sad anniversaries and manifest it in physical pain.

## External Events, Outside Influences, and Temporary Stress

These stressors come on every level, whether it be waiting the results of a medical exam, being trapped on the tarmac for hours, or interviewing for a new job. Most of the stress from these types of situations comes from feeling out of control: we can't rush the bloodwork, we can't make the plane move, and we have no sense of the hiring practices of a corporation.

Outside influences can also be a friend's problems that we are taking on. In essence, other people's emotions can make you sick. If your spouse is unemployed and having a hard time getting a job, his or her stress affects you. If a friend is a pessimist, his or her personality can become toxic for you. Ultimately, negative energy and emotions can impact both your daily routine as well as your health.

## Chronic Stress

Although most stress is caused by fleeting events, those who suffer from chronic stress feel as if there is no light at the end of the tunnel. This type of stress can arise from any number of events: a long-term illness, a dead-end job, a poor relationship, the list goes on. Sometimes people think they are finding relief from their stress at the bottom of a bottle or at the back of the refrigerator, but the only way to cope with significant stressors is to find positive ways to prevent it from becoming all-encompassing. Exercise, helping others (this works wonders in getting some people out of their self-pitying mood!), joining a support group or seeing a therapist can get you through a rough spot in your life.

Suffering from back pain can be incredibly stressful. You may wonder if you will ever be pain-free again and be able to do the things that you used to enjoy. The stress about your back pain often only increases the pain.

# THE TEN LAWS FOR YOUR BEST LIFE

Studies show that listening to soothing music 25 minutes per day can lower your stress hormone levels up to 25 percent, cutting your risk of back pain in half. Norwegian researchers prodded 500 people to exercise daily, and their risk of having back pain also dropped by 50 percent. Ultimately, there are just as many ways to help you manage the stress in your life as there are causes. Learning positive responses allows you to take charge and stay happier and healthier. In addition to the stress-relieving techniques that you will learn about in the next section, adopting the Ten Laws helps keep you in a mentally positive place. For the next three weeks (and beyond!), read these laws each morning. Keeping them at the forefront of your mind as you face your day will help you to stay positive and find small but healthier ways of coping with daily stressors.

### LAW 1: Take care of yourself.

Eat right and build in time for exercise. Give yourself time to rest. Think of things you love and make time for each one. Doing this allows you to feel good in your body and always have something enjoyable in your life.

### LAW 2: Build personal connections.

It's been shown that having friends helps us live longer! Social ties reduce our risk of disease by lowering blood pressure, heart rate, and cholesterol levels. It's important to give of ourselves to friends, as well as accept their help, support, and listening ears.

### LAW 3: Slow down.

Frequently a patient will speed-walk into my office, as if walking more quickly would let him or her get more done. Remember the song that goes, "Slow down, you move too fast/You got to make the mornin' last"? My patients always smile when I sing this to them. Maybe they are laughing at me, rather than with me, but it helps them remember one of my important prescriptions that is guaranteed to make you feel better: "Walk slower; drive slower; notice the passing scenery; take deep breaths; and make 'me' time." Although work, family and sleep take up much of our day, finding time for yourself helps your mind slow down and savor a part of the day. Part of slowing down involves learning to say no. By simplifying your schedule, you can bring your life into congruence. Incongruence results in stress, which causes back pain. If you don't stop the self-sabotage (whether it be indulging in that ice cream sundae when you need to lose weight or taking on too much), you will never feel better.

## LAW 4: Don't minimize the positives or maximize the negatives.

Feeling positive decreases stress, and positive feelings come from within. I often observe that women, particularly, are dismissive of their opportunities to shine. For example, if someone compliments a woman on a dress she's wearing, she is likely to respond with "This old thing?" or "I couldn't find anything else this morning." Men tend to grunt and brush aside comments as well.

Next time, instead of casting a compliment aside, nurture that positive view of yourself. Find self-confidence, which can help you find strength and resourcefulness in dealing with difficult times. It can also help you take negative feedback in stride. Instead of being crippled by criticism, use it as a motivator to become better!

## LAW 5: Let go.

Worrying is human nature but we should all spend less time doing it. The word "worry" comes from a Middle English word that means "to strangle" or "to choke." Worrying is actually a way we strangle ourselves. The best way to control your worrying is to recognize your concern and take three to five minutes to consider it. Have you prepared your child for his first walk home from school without you? Have you mentally prepared yourself for your new boss? If so, remind yourself that you have done everything you can, and that most things we worry about don't come to pass. If you don't have control over a situation, remind yourself of that and say to yourself, "If I can't control it, I won't sweat it." You'll be surprised at the number of situations that will improve once you realize this.

### LAW 6: Take a break.

Take a hot bath, plan a family vacation, or even turn off your phone while you eat dinner with your family. You will be amazed by how much better your back can feel if you just recharge your batteries.

### LAW 7: Recognize and acknowledge the problem.

Admitting you have a problem is the first step to healing. It isn't weak to admit you have a problem. The test of strength or weakness has to do with how you handle problems. Do you work to find a solution and improve yourself or do you let the problem get the better of you?

### LAW 8: Take action.

Consider what is happening that causes stress in your life and what approaches you could take to lessen the stress. Choose one and follow through. Remember, only you can help you. A friend, a self-help book, or a therapist can certainly give you advice, but you have to be willing to put advice into action and work. The early steps are generally small steps, but making small changes in your attitude can lead to big strides in the long-term.

### LAW 9: See the light at the end of the tunnel.

Stanford University performed a study and found out that mental outlook was the most effective way to predict future occurrences of back pain; it was even more accurate than a physical exam and an X ray. Remember that you can't undo certain events, but seeing beyond them can help change your physical reaction to them. Note any subtle ways in which you might already feel somewhat better as you deal with difficult situations.

### LAW 10: Take time to reflect.

Pausing to reflect can help provide you with perspective. Long walks, meditation or praying may help. Any solitary activity may well provide you with the opportunity to think things through.

We discussed the effect of relaxation of the muscles in the Structural Solutions, but back pain is so tightly linked to our emotional state that you can even raise the proverbial chicken-or-egg question: Which comes first, the pain or the distress about the pain? It's common for people who have severe back pain to suffer from mild depression. Although I typically favor a non-medication approach to treating back pain, I've noticed that some patients who start taking anti-depressants decrease their need for other pain medications:

Judi had been coming to us monthly for several years with complaints of chronic low back pain and overall stiffness. Regardless of the structural treatments we provided, Judi never felt better and resigned herself to the fact that it was just her nature to be tight and stiff due to her age and sedentary lifestyle. One day, when she came into the office for her monthly adjustment, she reported that she was completely pain-free. I asked what had caused such a remarkable improvement. She said she had been suffering from some mild depression, and her primary doctor had put her on some low level anti-depressants. The anti-depressant changed her life by banishing the tension she felt in her back.

Because a primary cause of back pain is emotional, it makes sense that an anti-depressant can have a profound impact on back pain. This doesn't mean you should try to obtain an anti-depressant if you don't really need it. Stress will happen throughout your entire life and developing positive emotional habits can help you build resilience and take care of yourself in hard times.

## HOW TO BUILD RESILIENCE

Resilience is the process of adapting well in the face of trauma, adversity, tragedy, threats, and other significant sources of stress and bouncing back from them. It's about facing challenges, changing what you can, and moving on. We all need this inner strength to cope with the ups and down of life. Here are four ways to build resilience:

### 1. MAINTAIN A HOPEFUL OUTLOOK.

Try to visualize what you want rather than worrying about what you fear. Studies on everything from heart disease to cancer

(continued on next page)

*(continued from previous page)*

show that a positive outlook can make a significant difference in survival rates. And remember, a predictor of back pain is emotional outlook. A positive outlook can spare you pain and just might save your life.

### 2. SET ACHIEVABLE GOALS.

Develop realistic goals, outline ways to achieve them, and each week, take one step toward one of your goals. Even if it seems like you aren't making much progress, you'll begin to see that small steps are leading you forward. When you begin moving in the direction you want to go, you feel empowered and less vulnerable.

### 3. WHAT DOESN'T KILL YOU MAKES YOU STRONGER.

Adversity sometimes has its benefits. Obviously, you would prefer to avoid it, but people often learn something about themselves or grow as a result of difficult times. They report a heightened appreciation for life with a renewed sense of self-worth, a more developed spirituality, better relationships, and a greater sense of strength as a result of what they lived through. Look for the silver lining and note your own personal growth in past situations. It will help you find strength in future ones.

### 4. GIVE BACK.

No matter how bad your stress, chances are someone else is worse off. Volunteering can give you some perspective and help you feel better about stressors in your life. You'll often see that people struggling even more than you have faith, hope, and spirit, which will help you find your own resilience.

## RELAXATION EXERCISES

All people, from the corporate CEO to the stay-at-home mom, are subject to stress. We can't always take a daily yoga class or a leisurely walk in the park to relax, so here are some quick exercises to help get you through the next hour, the next day, the next week . . .

### THE THINKER

Find a quiet spot—just close your office door if you have to! Sit in a comfortable pose, take off glasses if you wear them, and close your eyes. Press the fingertips of both hands lightly along the ridge above your brow. Take five slow breaths.

### DEEP BREATHING

What can be easier than this one? (It's actually not as easy as you think if you are stressed). The yogis know what they are doing when they place emphasis on "breath with motion." Just simply taking full, deep breaths, inhaling and exhaling completely, is extremely cleansing and calming. When people become stressed, their breathing rate speeds up, and in order to relax, the breath needs to be slowed down. All you have to do is:

► Inhale slowly for a count of 4.
► Hold it for a count of 4.
► Exhale for a count of 4.

Start by doing this exercise for two minutes. As you breathe, empty your mind of all thoughts. If they creep in, let them pass. Over time, try to extend the amount of time you devote to this practice.

### RELAXATION POSE

One of the most relaxing positions in yoga—and a method that can help migraines—involves lying on your back with your legs extended up the wall. Sitting with one hip aligned as close to the wall as possible, swing your legs up as you lie back so that both legs are extended up the wall and there is now

(continued on next page)

*(continued from previous page)*

space between your buttocks and the wall. Lie for 10 minutes, allowing blood to flow to the torso and the muscles along your spine to fully relax.

## WALKING

A study of back patients revealed that walking is not only a great stress reliever, but also helpful in relieving back pain. You don't have to power walk, but you should wear sensible footwear to keep your feet—and your back—in structurally sound positions.

# 14

## LOSE THE PAIN, GAIN ENERCHI

### MY THREE WEEK ENERCHI SOLUTION

Western medicine has become less and less personal. Today, we acknowledge that it's important for doctors to understand and treat, and not disregard the emotional root of physical pain. For the most part, stress does not change that much; there will always be work, traffic, illness, and even tragedy. But what can change is how your body handles the stress. I've found that Asian medicine tends to be more gentle and patient-centered, and that alone can be very healing. Learning to change your stress response by adopting certain relaxation practices can give you a greater sense of calm and control in what may otherwise have felt like unmanageable situations. I have seen some of my own patients benefit from acupressure, acupuncture, and the practice of Tai Chi, which led me to formulate my own Three Week Enerchi Solution based on Chinese philosophy. Just 21 days can help you release your tight muscles and change how you cope with life's frustrations and upsets.

### Change Your Chi

Stanford University's landmark study proved what I knew to be true: emotional outlook and stress is the number one factor for back pain. Still, when this study's results were released, I felt completely unprepared to help people who were suffering from back pain stemming from an emotional component. Offering solutions in my practice for only two-thirds of the problem (nutritional and structural) was unacceptable. I had to be able to offer a complete solution. I began to research Chinese medical philosophy, which is rooted in the belief that the body has a motivating energy that moves through a series of channels called meridians. This energy flow is called chi, which means life force.

The theory made sense to me: If we are feeling well, the energy flow is like a quickly flowing river with few detours. However, when we become stressed, this flow of energy gets blocked, throwing off our balance, or chi. This imbalance can lead to anything from irritability to serious pain.

Chinese medicine sees the cure to those muscles contractions that happen during periods of stress is to get the chi flowing again. Eastern doctors use acupressure and acupuncture to unblock the chi and recommend diet and exercise (such as Tai Chi) to maintain balance once it is righted again.

Your daily experiences, both negative and positive, affect your chi. When you listen to the morning news about terror threats, murders, house fires, and other tragedies, your chi is negatively affected. When you listen to classical music and take a brisk walk, your chi is positively affected. The way we react to different experiences also affects our chi. The example I always use is eating ice cream. If you are eating a hot fudge sundae to celebrate an accomplishment, it can positively affect your chi. However, eating a sundae when you are bored or depressed about your weight will have the opposite effect. I once prescribed a ski vacation to a patient who came in complaining of terrible lower back pain. After a full examination and consideration of all his issues, I surmised his pain stemmed from difficult political issues at his office. I told him, "Go on. Get out of here. Go skiing, slowly at first, but you'll be fine!" And he was. Getting away from work stress and doing what he loved was curative.

The essence of this lesson is that you need to improve the aspects of your life that are negatively affecting your chi and make time for things that positively affect your inner energy. These solutions are unique to you.

# TAI CHI

Tai Chi Chuan originated in China as one of the martial arts. It involves dozens of postures and gestures performed in sequence. Tai Chi cleanses the body's tissue of accumulated stress, boosting all aspects of our health systems. Today, it is most often considered a low-impact series of flowing movements that take the body through positions of energy balance. You do comparable moves in yoga.

Tai Chi boosts the immune system and reduces incidence of depression, anxiety, and chronic pain. It increases mental relaxation and allows blood pressure to drop. Practiced over a period of time, an individual can become more relaxed, gain better balance and greater concentration, and increase his or her conscious circulation of vital energy through the body. This relaxation response happens because Tai Chi Chuan and other Chinese exercises involve systematic mental programs of mood and mood training.

## TAI CHI YOUR PAIN AWAY

Here are a few simple Tai Chi exercise for you to try at home!

## HUGGING THE TREE

Stand in an alert but relaxed position with your knees slightly bent, feet shoulder-width apart, hands at your sides. Breathe in and out slowly for ten repetitions, allowing your mind to become clear and calm. Now raise your arms as if you were hugging a big round tree and hold this position as you breathe normally for about 30 seconds, visualizing the flow of energy between your hands. Shake out your arms and repeat three more times. This is a good way to help your chi flow throughout your body.

## AWAKEN THE CHI

Stand with your feet shoulder-width apart and parallel, toes pointing straight out. Stand tall, shoulders relaxed, your gaze straight out ahead of you. Let your arms hang loosely at your sides, fingers curved naturally with the palms facing your body.

*(continued on next page)*

*(continued from previous page)*

Tuck in your tailbone and breathe out as you let your body sink down, allowing your knees to bend slightly. Breathe in as you rise up and draw your arms up to shoulder height, palms facing down, elbows and wrists slightly bent. Turn your hands so the palms face out to the front, keeping your fingers curved naturally.

Breathe out as you draw your arms back down to your sides with the palms facing to the back and sink into the knees. Breathe in and raise your body up and stand with your palms facing your thighs. Repeat this sequence three times.

### An Open Mind for the Alternatives: My Personal Awakening to the Power of Tapping

The Chinese philosophy of Tai Chi led to me to search for what else we can do to obtain inner balance and rid ourselves of emotional back pain. I attended my first lecture by Dr. James Durlacher, who wrote a book called *Freedom from Fear Forever*, based on the studies of Roger Callahan, PhD., and his "five minute phobia cure." Callahan appeared on national television and literally cured people of their fear within five minutes. People who could not even look at a snake would be holding them just a few minutes later. At Durlacher's lecture, he was looking for volunteers to demonstrate his work. I had been suffering from an irrational fear of flying and though I found the "quick cure" unlikely, I volunteered. Dr. Durlacher had me visualize myself flying, and I started to feel those pre-flight nerves kicking in. He then began tapping different points that he explained were acupressure points. In just three minutes, I felt calmer about flying, and to my extreme surprise, on the flight home, my anxiety, sweaty palms, and uncomfortable stomach all went away.

I was intrigued. I had been skeptical of Durlacher's alternative therapy, and yet it worked. A patient then told me about a technique that he experienced called Neuro Emotional Technique (NET), and my father and I went to Atlanta to see what it was all about. NET was created to deal with emotional tension that becomes manifested into physical pain rather than being extinguished in the body. This technique is based on the acupuncture circuitry of the Chinese, who, thousands of years ago, found that specific meridians or pathways correlate with specific emotions. For example, the kidney meridian relates to fear and the lung meridian relates to grief. It was then discovered that the specific meridian pathways related to specific points on the spine. By treating these specific spinal points while contacting the correlating meridian points, you could eliminate tension and stress spots. Once again, this technique almost seemed unbelievable to me until NET was done on me. In just a few minutes, the tension in my neck and shoulder literally melted away. This was the second time that I had been treated with tapping, and in both times I felt much less discomfort.

## Why Acupressure and Acupuncture Work

Traditional Chinese medicine distinguishes between the mind and the body, and their restorative methods of acupressure and acupuncture are curative for both somatic (of the body) and psychological disorders.

The flow of chi can be blocked at a variety of points in the human body, many of which have direct correlation to points on the spine. Most practitioners today act on at least 600 points, spaced relatively evenly over the entire body. Stimulation may be made by hand (massotherapy or acupressure) or needles (acupuncture), as well as heat (moxibustion).

## Acupressure

During a good massage, you are awake, but will feel some sleep-like qualities and will leave in a completely different state of relaxation. The massage itself has completely changed your chi. You can easily start out by doing a self-help method of acupressure on yourself!

### TRY IT YOURSELF!
### GOLF BALL ACUPRESSURE

Using a reflexology ball or even a golf ball, sit down in a comfortable chair and take off your shoes. Place the golf ball on the floor and rest your foot on top of the ball. Roll the ball under your foot from heel to arch to toes in a circular motion for a couple of minutes. Repeat on the other foot. The ball puts pressure on the acupressure points in your foot, helping to relax your entire body—a practice also known as reflexology.

## Acupuncture

Acupuncture involves the insertion of fine needles along the meridians to reestablish energy flow, restore balance, and encourage healing. The needles are left in place for approximately 40 minutes, and they may be manipulated by hand by the practitioner or stimulated with electricity. The needle creates a dull ache, tingling or numbness (known as *de qi*) as the energy flow is reopened, and while this sounds painful, you will feel only a little pinch and then it becomes actually quite relaxing!

Acupuncture works on the belief that a web of connective tissue supports our body's organs and other tissues. The needles are typically inserted into points where connective tissues bundle together, often around the joints. When the needle is inserted into the tissue, endorphins are released. A small inflammatory response is triggered, causing physiological changes. It is speculated that the process of the small sting of the needle may prohibit passage of stronger pain signals, which is one of the reasons why acupuncture is successful!

Acupuncture does come with slight risk of bruising and infection, so it's important to get a referral from your doctor and make certain you are working with a licensed practitioner.

# THREE WEEK ENERCHI SOLUTION

After exploring acupressure, acupuncture and other relaxation techniques, particularly the protocol and practice of Gary Craig's Emotional Freedom Technique (EFT) which allows anyone to stimulate their own tapping points, and Dr. Scott Walker's NET, I was certain you could alter the stress response and eliminate the tension in your body via acupressure points. I went on to become certified in NET and formulated my own treatment. My Three Week Enerchi Balancing Plan allows you to relax your tight muscles, rejuvenate your energy, and balance your chi. I understand that many of you may be skeptical about what sounds like a New Age concept but it's important that I discuss these options. Many of my patients have found similar relief from their emotional back pain using these methods. If you think that your back pain may be stress-related, I encourage you to open your mind and try it. While you may look and feel a bit silly, it will help relax you, thereby allowing your tight, contracted muscles to release and ease pain. It only takes three weeks to feel a difference and you certainly won't be any worse off!

## Tap the Stress Out

My Three Week Enerchi Solution involves a combination of tapping and breathing to help you maximize your relaxation and regain your inner balance. Tapping has become quite popular in helping people with a myriad of health issues, not just back pain. I understand that it looks crazy, but it certainly worked for me and can make a big difference for you. For the next three weeks, do the breathing/tapping sequence three times a day, in the morning, at mid-day, and in the evening. Here are the steps to follow:

### Two-Minute Breathing

Bring your hands to your forehead. Inhale for five seconds, hold for five seconds, and exhale for five seconds. Repeat eight times or for two minutes.

### Tapping Protocol

I have modified the tapping technique by combining the work of Dr. Durlacher with that of Gary Craig, and my plan offers simple self-help. There are ten points to tap on the body, including two on each hand. You should be able to run through an entire sequence in about two minutes!

#### THE TEN TAPPING POINTS

1. eyebrow
2. side of eye
3. under eye
4. under nose
5. chin
6. collarbone
7. under arm
8. top of head
9. side of wrist (karate chop)
10. wrist between fourth and fifth fingers

Before starting, identify your stressor and grade your level of unease. Begin tapping. At each point, tap for ten seconds while you do each of the following: close your eyes, open your eyes, look up, look down, look down and to the right, look down and to the left, rotate your eyes clockwise, and then counter clockwise, hum a verse of "Happy Birthday" and count to ten. This process seemingly engages different aspects of the brain. After running through the sequence, evaluate how you feel about the stress. You should find that it has decreased.

After each protocol of breathing and tapping you should feel more relaxed and energized. You can also check your flexibility before and after; you should find it improved after your muscles have released!

Remember, consistency is key, so commit to the tapping and breathing for three weeks before you give up. The changes may be small to start, so monitor your progress. You'll likely find that by the end of the three weeks, a big change (which you may not have noticed day-to-day) has occurred!

. . .

IT'S THE MOST *amazing, uplifting feeling of physical lightness when Dr. Sinett practices his method of tapping down my spine. I would never have believed how powerful an effect this would have on my body, releasing all tension and stress in a matter of minutes. There's just no other form of therapy for me. As a mother of two young children, a wife, and full-time professional (running a firm with 40 staffers), I am exposed to stress on a daily basis. Unfortunately, I'm not good at letting this go myself and as a result, it holds in my upper body (back, neck and shoulders). Yet, this is magically released when I visit Dr. Sinett. This release of the stress rolls into the emotional aspects of my life in the most positive way. It's such an empowering treatment. Living without pain and discomfort, coupled with maintaining strength in my upper body, allows me to be confident in myself. This is incredibly valuable, as I pass this confidence along to my children and all other people around me in life!*

*Nadia Biski*

## ANOTHER ALTERNATIVE: BIOFEEDBACK

In my office, we do something called biofeedback, a non-invasive method that measures your nervous system's response to stress by tracking skin temperature, respiration, muscle tension and heart rate. The patient then performs specific relaxation and breathing exercises, sometimes via relaxation CD, that teach you how to positively affect these biological processes. Athletes use biofeedback to help them get in the "zone." If you are interested in learning more biofeedback, you can start by downloading two inexpensive apps that the biofeedback counselor in my practice recommends: Breathe2relax and Yoga Nidra.

# 15

# WHO TO SEE FOR EMOTIONAL ISSUES

While you will find that the tapping, breathing, and other relaxation and coping strategies will help you feel less tense, more in control and at peace, and free from pain, sometimes you need an unbiased third party to listen and offer advice, especially during a time of particular stress. While I consider Level 1 Emotional Care the appropriate starting place, here are the doctors you can see when helping yourself requires help from someone else.

**Level 2:** A counselor, therapist, or biofeedback specialist can help you work through your stress, gain perspective, and offer additional coping and emotional healing techniques.

**Level 3:** A psychiatrist is trained in how emotions can impact your health and back and can prescribe medications to help with emotional back pain. Studies have shown that anti-depressants have worked better than anti-inflammatories, which makes sense given that emotions are the number one cause of back pain! While I like to encourage non-medication alternatives, sometimes medicine is necessary.

# THE THREE-WEEK TOTAL TAKE-AWAY

## Three Easy Tips to Help You Target Your Emotional Solution

The tips in this section are designed to help you fix the little things. And little things added up make a big difference.

### 1. Just Breathe.

Inhale for five seconds, hold for five seconds, and exhale for five seconds. Repeat eight times, or for two minutes.

### 2. Tap Away.

My quick tapping protocol will stimulate your enerchi and make you feel less uptight and less anxious, creating a physical reaction in your body allowing those contracted muscles to release and relax.

### 3. Meditate.

Meditation allows you to reign in your mind and your worries. Listen to a meditation track that talks you through a relaxing exercise to release the back tension that may have built up during the day. Performing this every night will help you manage your emotions and pain!

# 16

## THE TOTAL TAKE-AWAY

### Three Weeks to Three-Tiered Success

### 1. It is all related!

This is what I call the home run principle: your body is interconnected and all of the three factors (structural, digestive, and emotional) are interrelated. If you are exercising, you will notice your workouts feel better when you choose proper fuel. If you are eating healthier food, your moods are going to improve. If your moods are better, you are going to be carrying less tension and feel better. By impacting one factor you are impacting the other two. Remember, your spine is a shoelace and when one area of your body is off kilter, you feel it in your back. In order to be back pain-free, you need to have balance in all three key aspects. The principles to getting your back functioning great are the same exact principles for your overall health and well-being!

### 2. Listen to your body.

As we've learned, the body speaks a language, talking to you via pain, bowel movements, moods, etc. Ignoring the signs of your body only means more pain, so listen closely, respond immediately, and be consistent. Start looking at your shoes, noting the purchase date of your mattress, and cleaning out your heavy purse so that you are being proactive and preventing your body from crying out in pain in the first place!

### 3. Three weeks forms a habit.

Three weeks is all it takes to create a new habit. Three weeks can go by pretty slowly when you are trying to wean yourself off caffeine or sugar or get yourself to the gym, but soon, your body will ask for that water or that workout, and you won't even miss what you gave up. In the long run, three weeks is a very short period of time to allow you to be free from pain at the end!

# ACKNOWLEDGMENTS

This section is truly the hardest to write because properly acknowledging everyone who was instrumental in this book is literally impossible. I feel like a famous actor running way too long in their acceptance speech.

This entire journey started when my father, a practicing Chiropractor, was stricken with severe back pain that incapacitated him for nine months. It was Dr. George Goodheart who had the convictions and beliefs to examine my father differently than anyone else had. Dr. Goodheart determined that my father's severe back pain was caused by poor diet and an inflamed digestive system. This discovery became a pivotal moment in my family's life and inspired my father's and my life's work.

Practicing alongside my father for about 10 years really was the most wonderful experience of my life. While I never felt I grasped all of his teachings, I am forever grateful for all that I absorbed. Everyday I go to the office, with my father's water mug and giant picture of his smiling face, and do my best to help as many people as possible.

I want to thank my mother for always supporting me and being the rock of the family. She has never once complained since my father's passing. They say that one's true character comes out when adversity strikes, and my mother is a true testament to love and resiliency.

I also want to thank my beautiful wife and kids. My daughter, Taylor, the true author in the family, has made me so proud by publishing two children's books (A *Weasel on an Easel* and *Jack on a Plaque*) and donating all of the *proceeds to charity*. I want to thank my son, Kyle, who seems to have inherited the "Todd gene" and a love to hang out in the office with only minor damage. I also want to thank my wife for being the best wife a guy could ever have and for the support and freedom to write this book.

To the actual writing of the book, I want to encourage anyone who has an idea for a book to get to it. Believe me, if I can write a book anyone can. The reason is that there are plenty of professional people who can help! I want to thank Jayne Pillemer, my writer and editor. She has the amazing ability to take every decent idea or thought that I have and turn it into something legible and intelligent. She also has the ability to take every not so great idea that I have and edit it out gracefully. I'm also so grateful to David Zanes for the fantastic photos and to Alex Torres for being a great fitness model.

I want to thank Willow Jarosh of C and J Nutrition for all of her wonderful writing, recipes and ideas throughout the Digestive section. Please check out her book and writings at cjnutrition.com. Thank you to my literary agent, Cathy Hemming, who believed in me from the beginning, as well as my publisher, Pauline Neuwirth, the head of East End publishing. I also want to thank Krupp Kommunications for taking me on as a client and doing their part to spread the word about The Sinett Solution. I also want to thank my coworkers at Midtown Integrative Health and Wellness. They truly are the most talented people I know, and it is an absolute pleasure to be able to work side by side with them. Thank you especially to Tasman Rubel for coordinating the practice, which is an enormous undertaking.

A special thank you to my patients. To be able to meet and help so many wonderful people has been a complete blessing. Because of them I have never "worked" a day in my life, and this book comes from direct communication from all of the people who have walked through my practice door. They have served as my test subjects and helped me produce truly valuable findings.

Lastly, I want to thank you, the reader, who may now be open to new concepts and ideas. One of the greatest gifts in life is to be able to pass on information. This book is a culmination of many people's efforts, and I hope that you can benefit from this information. My wish for you is that you will have a better back in just three weeks!

*Dr. Todd Sinett*

# How Much Do You *Really* Know About Back Pain?

Answer Key

**1.** Back pain is the second leading cause of missed work days. Only the common cold causes more employee absence.

**2. E: Two of the above:** mildly helpful and potentially harmful in diagnosing back pain. MRIs are effective in uncovering serious medical problems such as tumors or infections; however when it comes to back pain, MRIs often provide the doctor with only localized information, which can lead to higher rates of medical intervention without better long-term results.

**3. B: False. Your back is a lot stronger than you think!** If you bend down to pick up something and your back gives out, it is very rarely because you bent the wrong way, and more likely is the result of a build-up of other bad habits, like poor nutrition!

**4. D: Two of the above, B and C.** The role of diet is the most overlooked cause of back pain. Anything that can cause digestive distress can affect the muscular system resulting in back pain. Essentially too much of any-thing—even salad—is not a good thing! If you think your diet could be causing your back pain, check out Section 2.

**5. C: Sit-ups and crunches work an abdominal muscle called the rectus abdominis, which has no stabilizing factor on the back.** Essentially, you are exercising the wrong muscle! The best abdominal exercise to stabilize the back is an exercise called a skinny that works the transversus abdom-inis. It's simple, and it strengthens your core in the right way. All you have to do is this: Exhale all of your breath while pulling your navel in and up and hold for 10 seconds.

**6. B: False. There are thousands of people who have a disc herniation but have absolutely no symptoms.** In a landmark study published in the *New England Journal of Medicine,* researchers ran MRIs on 98 people who never had back pain, and 28% of those people showed a disc herniation. BUT if you do suffer from pain from a disc herniation, a non-invasive structural treatment, like using my Backbridge™ twice a day for two minute intervals, can help relieve your pain!

**7. D: Each back pain case is unique.** There is no one right answer for everyone, and remember that the successful treatment and diagnosis of back pain could be a combination of things!

**8. A: An over-simplified model.** Yes, putting on additional weight can cause strain on your back, but remember, your back is strong! The correlation of weight has more to do with the unhealthy eating and lifestyle habits, which cause digestive-induced pain, than the physical load of the additional weight.

**9. D:** Surgery can be the greatest blessing for someone suffering from back pain; however, the overall results for back surgery are not that good. In a long range study, researchers found that people who had back surgery felt better quicker, but 5 and 10 years later, the people who underwent surgery compared to the people who did not have surgery had similar results.

**10. A: True. 85% of people will suffer from back pain, and 85% of people don't exercise regularly.** Proper exercise is one of the most important things you can do to prevent and relieve back pain. However, always listen to your body. Exercise should feel good. If something hurts, don't do it!

**11. B:** Stanford University studied 3,000 Boeing employees for more than four years and found stress and emotional outlook were the most important predictor and factor for future back pain than any physical measure.

**12. D:** According to recent data, the yearly expenditure for the diagnosis and treatment of back pain is approximately $80 billion.

**13. C:** The worst posture while sitting is slouched forward, but sitting up tall can also put too much of a compressive load on your back. The best way to sit is to lean back at a 135 degree angle. Get a desk chair that extends back and when traveling, use every opportunity to recline your seat. Every hour get up and move around—our bodies were not built for sitting all day!

**14. A:** There are three factors to back pain:
1. Your structural system (muscles and bones)
2. Your diet and nutrition
3. Your emotions and stress

Balancing these three aspects is the key to staying back problem-free. Working on only two of these things won't do it! Pain can only be cured by targeting all points in the triad!

**15. E: All of the above.** Yes, back pain can be the sign of a more significant health issue, but for the most part back pain is your body's attempt to tell you that something is wrong. For many people, back pain is just a sign of unhealthy habits, and changing these unhealthy habits into healthy ones can impact your life in many more ways than just back pain. Back pain can be a great gift if it helps you achieve a more balanced life!

---

Now that you have the fast answers, it's time to learn the Sinett Solution to bettering your back in just three weeks!

# THE DOCTOR'S PRODUCT PICKS

Many patients ask me what I specifically do to keep myself free of back pain and healthy. My response is two-part:

1. Prevention is always better than needing intervention.
2. If you do have back pain, you want to learn from it and get rid of it.

This learning means paying attention to all structural, nutritional, and emotional causes and using products and methods that can improve your body and mind. There are many different products that I recommend that can be part of your total solution.

Here are my product picks for structurally-caused pain:

---

### For SLEEP:

► **Chiroflow Water Pillow**

*The #1 recommended chiropractic pillow. Water-filled pillows are dynamic and ensure ideal neck posture while you sleep!*

www.chiroflow.com

---

### For ORTHODICS:

► **Foot Levelers Orthodics**

*Feet, gait, and posture are different for everyone, which is why I love these functional orthodics that are individually created for each patient. They help straighten posture to relieve back pain.*

www.footlevelers.com

► **WalkFit**

*These comfortable orthodics have cushioning and shock absorption and help realign your spine and pelvis to reduce knee, hip, and back pain.*

www.walkfit.com

## For PAIN RELIEF:

▶ **Trumedic Tens Unit**

*TENS (Transcutaneous Electrical Nerve Stimulation) therapy is clinically proven to relieve a range of pains, including muscle tension. Trumedic makes a great unit for personal use.*

www.trumedic.com

▶ **BioFreeze**

*Biofreeze is the #1 clinically recommended topical analgesic to relieve pain. It is less bulky than ice, doesn't smell and is really easy to use. Biofreeze is great for sore muscles; easing back, shoulder, and neck pain; and reducing painful joints. Available in gel, roll-on, and spray.*

www.biofreeze.com

▶ **Mueller Lumbar Back Brace**

*The double layer design of this brace allows for custom fit and adjustable compression to the abdomen and lower back to help give your relief from injuries, spasms, and strenuous activity. The fabric is comfortable for all-day wear!*

www.muellersportsmed.com/archive/back_brace_lumbar.htm

## For the JAW:

▶ **ProTeeth Mouthguard**

*If you clench your teeth, a mouthguard can help prevent jaw pain from grinding. I like ProTeeth mouth guards because they are custom molded and can be ordered online.*

www.proteethguard.com

## For the BACK/CORE:

▶ **Backbridge**

*I created it, and I can't recommend it enough! It works for so many different symptoms by realigning your posture and counteracting forward flexion, which leads to core imbalance.*

www.backbridge.com

Now for Nutrition. In my No More Back Pain diet, you learned that fruit should be eaten alone and, therefore, makes a great snack. But I know everyone wants other snack options. And you should always make sure you have a satiating snack so that you keep your blood sugar from dropping and keep yourself from getting too hungry and overeating at your next meal. Here are my favorite stay-with-you snacks and food products:

▶ **Bear Naked Granola**—I loved Bear Naked Granola for a crunchy snack that comes in lots of flavors, many with nuts for a protein punch! A selection of their granolas can be found on their website: https://www.bearnaked.com/en_US/fuel-up.html

▶ **Kashi Cereals**—I love these cereals, especially the GOLEAN versions, which have a ton of protein and fiber to keep you full until dinner. I find the little clusters as poppable as popcorn! Kashi cereals can be found at https://www.kashi.com/our-foods/cold-cereal/kashi-golean-crunch-cereal.

▶ **Stonyfield Organic Yogurt**—I try to buy organic where I can, and Stonyfield Organic makes delicious plain and vanilla yogurts (which are lower in sugar than the fruited yogurts). I opt for the Greek versions, which are higher in protein. They are delicious topped with berries, nuts, or even a drizzle of maple syrup. I also love making a small smoothie with fruit and yogurt combined to help me power through my afternoons. Stonyfield offers products and recipes on their website at http://www.stonyfield.com.

And finally, are there products to help stress and bad emotions? The answer is a resounding yes. You now know my tapping technique, the power of tai chi and positive thinking, but in addition to these things, I also have found a great support system in Edwige Gilbert, a wellness and stress management coach. I recommend everyone visit her website, newlifedirections.com, for additional techniques that might help you recenter and stay mentally and spiritually healthy. Edwige offers group meetings, personalized meditation CDs, and a Victory Contract, among other things, to help get you and keep you on track.

One World Academy (oneworldacademy.com) is a school of wisdom that embraces the similarities of all humans. Their site offers meditations and podcasts to help everyone recenter and live with purpose and fulfillment. I've encountered many who have benefited from their meditation tracks!

# INDEX